The Unicorn Wellness Handbook

Tips & tactics from the practical to the magical
to invoke your most magical self inside and out

Tandy Gutierrez

This book is dedicated to my grandmother, Cleta Mitchell.

Ammie, I know you are with me every step of the way along my unicorn path. You modeled behaviors of self-care and spiritual ritual long before I ever knew what the terms were. I promise to do my very best to model and teach self-loving practices to as many as the universe sees fit.

Thank you for being a guide to me in this life and the next.

Table of Contents

HOW TO FEED A UNICORN

The Reset

The Reset Menu

Dear Unicorns~

I'm a unicorn.
I want you to be one too.
You are a glorious unicorn.
You just haven't learned the steps to
invoke her yet.

I'm here to facilitate your unicorn
transformation.
I'm here to say "I love you! I see you!
You're wonderful and magical!"
I'm here to say "You don't get to be
mundane anymore. It's time to be a
unicorn!"

Unicorns symbolize the most powerful and
pure magic available in the universe.

When you are a unicorn you automatically
engage in active pursuit of your dreams.
When you are a unicorn you put yourself
on a high-speed train to successful,
positive evolution.

Unicorns are all about magical
manifestation of body, mind, and spirit.

The universe is rooting for you to show up as your best self for the greatest good of all involved.

Miracles happen.
Expect miracles.
Accept miracles.

In order to trip the wire on your personal miracle you'll need to meet the universe halfway by invoking your inner unicorn.

Unicorns create massive positive change in the world and my purpose is to nurture and invoke as many as possible across the globe, in order to make the world a better, more empowered, divinely unique, and sparkling place.

This handbook teaches you the steps to becoming a unicorn through movement, fuel, self-care, and spiritual ritual.

What is a Unicorn?

Unicorns symbolize infinite hope and unlimited potential. In traditional mythology unicorns only reveal themselves to those who are pure of heart. Unicorns, once revealed, are capable of bestowing true healing upon the pure of heart (keep in mind the definition of healing is *to make better*) … basically, once you've discovered a unicorn, you have the opportunity to invoke its magic for yourself. When you invoke the power of your own inner unicorn, you make everything better simply by existing.

Becoming a unicorn is a magical ripple effect in this 3D reality.

Unicorns are capable of shifting from the earthly plane to the spirit world — it's as simple as walking out your front door and back in. They balance the real-deal living of life with the cosmic knowing of the universe. In other words, they pay their bills, go to work, exercise, feed themselves with the cleanest fuel they can, and all the while they keep an equal portion of themselves anchored in the ethers through meditation, essential oils, tarot, and crystals. They remember that they are children of God, made of stardust and never separate from the infinite magic of love and momma earth and the divine cosmos. Unicorns walk in silent strength because they know where they came from and who they are.

Unicorns take things at their own pace. They head down a consistent path to health with a connection to the divine. Unicorns balance full, busy lives with sweet, calm, and kind nurturing habits. Unicorns listen to their gut and connect deeply and daily with their intuition; your very own internal, innate magic. Unicorns approach their days, weeks, and years with hope and potential — undistracted and unencumbered by imbalances in the body, mind, and spirit.

You are a unicorn. You are a magical gift to the universe capable of successes even you can't imagine…… accessible once you activate and share your true unicorn self by honoring this human experience and tending to the body and life you have been given.

Unicorns take up space in the world as a ball of glowing rainbow energy. Unicorns are fearless. They are not afraid to be themselves and ditch what anyone else says or thinks of them or what the cultural norms say they need or should be. They never put on effects or pretend; they don't have to. Unicorns are deeply rooted in momma earth, in themselves, in love, and in doing. They make their mark on the world.

Unicorns sparkle, and shine because that's who they are. They are powerful. They are loving, genuine, willing to get in the dirt and work while also allowing the infinite wisdom of the universe to guide them to and through the unknown. Unicorns are fearless because they know they are always supported by the universe. Even and especially when the earthly experience is difficult, ugly, and upended.

Unicorns show up and change everything for the better, simply by being present. Their energy alchemizes their environment.

Unicorns embody the wisdom that allows them to see past false paradigms, illusions, lies, and antiquated rhetoric. They are in constant evolution towards the better with a connection of intellect, intuition, and love that is unstoppable.

It's time to transform into your most empowered, unique self, inside and out. It's time to participate consciously in your own evolution. It's time to participate in a wellness revolution because personal growth is the most important process of this incarnation. You should never feel like the person you were a year, five years, 10 or 20 years ago.....The universe wants you to be more evolved, more educated, more balanced, more capable, full of sparkle and shine, and flat out better!

It's Time to be a Unicorn

The Unicorn Wellness Handbook is a call to action. It's a wake-up call doused in glitter to remind you you're here on this planet to sparkle and shine. You're here to heal.

Healing may have always sounded like woo-woo magic, but it's not about magically *poof*ing away all the hurts, disappointments, challenges, anger, and frustration. Healing is one of my favorite words because the actual definition of "heal" is *to make better.* To lessen the aches and pains. To transform our deepest hurts into our greatest strengths and our highest magic.

Healing means ditching the hurt, as excuses, to keep you from evolving for the better. Healing means becoming fearless (doing things in spite of fear). Healing means living this life to its most magical capacities. Healing means pushing the edges of possibility and harnessing hope so that you can be of greatest service to as many as possible. Healing is about giving your gifts and showing up as your best you.

We are all here to make things better in both tiny and mighty ways and the truth of the matter is all we can ever change is ourselves and by evolving for the better, we actually make the world a better place, one unicorn at a time.

When you become a unicorn you learn to show up in the world as your best self. Unicorns shine like only those who live with a balance of heart and intellect can. Each person that invokes their inner unicorn literally makes the world a better place.

Healing = bettering.
By healing yourself you make the world a better place.

The Handbook

The Unicorn Wellness Handbook focuses on lifestyle habits, rituals, and practices that craft a #lifebydesign and allow *you* to make decisions that are a fit for *your* best life. I focus on the things that can truly make you feel like you sparkle and shine every day (or at least a greater average than not, because let's be honest … we are actually human and we all have low, difficult, down days). The goal of this handbook is for you to have tools that make you feel empowered on the greater average of days AND be more capable of handling the crazy, unexpected life that can come at us (daily).

I teach you the tactics and tools to be a unicorn. I get to teach them because I know clearly and deeply what it feels like when you don't sparkle and shine in full unicorn grandeur — when your inner unicorn is buried so deep you don't even know it's there.

I've been through it all: crazy schedules; constant travel; chronic health issues; multiple moves across the country; marriage; divorce; marriage again; running businesses; answering to others for everything; answering to no one; pregnancies; births; a miscarriage; a stepchild that took time to bond with; unschooling my littles; world schooling;

divorced parents; being an adoptee; a father who went to federal prison when I was 13; a highly abusive, suicidal mother; sexual assault as a child; medical battles that turned into legal battles with my oldest son when he was three months old; three autoimmune diseases; a thyroidectomy; and a hip repair. The loss of a father, and the loss of the mother who raised me.

Life is messy and the lessons of life can be deep and incredibly painful, but if I can be a unicorn — if I can transform despite a litany of reasons to genuinely not evolve, succeed, or feel wanted and worthy — so can you.

Learning to invoke your inner unicorn allows for healing, both shallow and deep. Learning to invoke your inner unicorn offers you sweetness in a world of mess. Becoming a unicorn allows for the hope of the innocent child to return in full glory. Becoming a unicorn takes time, effort, and doing. It takes some work. I didn't evolve overnight. I'm ever-evolving. I'm still doing it. But had I known these steps, if I had access to them as I'm offering them up to you, I would have evolved sooner and smoother. As a magical creature in a mundane world, I would have suffered less.

I want less suffering for you.

This handbook gives you solid tools you can embrace, practice, and run with. You'll have these tools to go back to anytime you need. Because, let's be honest, being a unicorn is an ongoing evolution. Being a unicorn takes practice. Being a unicorn requires repetition and time. Practicing the tactics and techniques in this handbook allow you to harness the healing power of your inner unicorn.

My hope is that my personal journey serves to help smooth and expedite yours.

Why I Teach

I wrote this handbook because it continues to blow me away how many people feel downright terrible day-to-day. I want to scoop everyone up in a motherly hug and tell them everything's going to be okay — and here's how we're going to put the pieces back together. We all need structure combined with magic and whimsy to get to our best self. Balance is the key to all things. True sparkle and shine comes from knowing when to push and when to pull, when to celebrate, when to play, and when to buckle down … and sometimes we need a real deal momma to snatch us up by an ear and put us on a structured path to the magical goods of a life evolved.

For nearly two decades I have taught wellness because I used to be one of those people who accepted feeling *off* as the norm. I had belly issues, chronic fatigue, bouts of depression, cystic acne, and anxiety that eventually became full blown panic attacks. I saw multiple credible doctors and practitioners and was told that I was simply "stressed" and needed antidepressants. I wished for a handbook for my own body and felt like no one was teaching wellness or fitness in a straightforward manner. I wanted real answers with real methods of improvement from both medical and alternative sides of the health table and I was happy (still am) to aim for *better* because not only does "perfect" not exist, when you feel so very low and terrible, better is down right magical.

I never did find one linear path towards my inner sparkle and shine. I didn't feel heard or understood and I certainly didn't feel empowered to heal. I did learn to become my own best advocate. For 12 years I sifted through research, reading, and trial and error, that has culminated in my best health to date and turned it all into clear techniques and habits to create healing in others. My path to healing rode in on a unicorn, in my personal experiences and intuition. I refused to listen to the *intellectual chatter* and I fiercely warriored for my own magic, inner knowing and gut instincts.

I'm here to give you the true gift of becoming a unicorn; that gift is rooted deeply in your inner knowledge, your instincts ... your intuition.

To invoke the strength of your inner unicorn, your deep knowing without linear proof, you have to peel the layers of your human experience, like an onion, complete with the tears, to get to the unicorn waiting for you at the center.

Your unicorn is waiting. It's already there. It has always been there. It's time to let it out.

My Unicorn Invocation

Truth be told I've had multiple unicorn transformations in my life. I hope to have more. Since we are ever-evolving and always becoming more and never less than we are, there is always another level. There are always challenges that present themselves to facilitate our learning. Every challenge is an opportunity to learn and every illness is an opportunity to heal.

Before I can teach you how to be a unicorn it's important that you know my story, how I became a unicorn. My story is one of my functional, physical health. It's what truly led me to write this handbook.

Before I was a Unicorn

From the age of 18 I had thyroid nodules that kept multiplying. I had chronic fatigue, anxiety, panic attacks, chronic sinus infections, acne, mysterious belly bloating, gas, pain, and let's just say it, chronic diarrhea.

I went to doctors and I went to therapists. I went to every alternative practitioner I could find or afford and they all basically told me I was 'stressed.' Um. Okaaaaay. Seriously? Yes, I was a living, working person in the world but I loved the things I did and at my gut level I knew that was not the culprit. I didn't accept their answers. Ever. I didn't even accept it when they handed me antidepressants. I was busy but internally happy and thought, "This is baloney. I don't feel well but not because my *head* is wrong. Something in my belly is causing the veil I feel covering my vibrancy." My sparkle and shine had a heavy curtain over it and I wasn't willing to blow off the potential to heal from the inside out. Because, let's be real, no one knows your body as well as you and nothing is stronger than your intuition, your knowing, your connection to the divine, higher self … to your inner unicorn. I was convinced it was food and self-care related and embarked on any and all variations of food, and wellness regimes I could. God bless my husband who stood by me at each variation and step. It was not easy on me but no easier on him as I tried protocol after protocol.

From ages 18 to 32 I had periods of time I was healthier on the inside but I was never *well*. I always required more recovery time than the people I was surrounded by. Some symptoms just never went away. Panic attacks, anxiety, acne, and diarrhea were still the kickers. I just *managed* them, I didn't address them and I just quit discussing or thinking about my internal health. I figured if I looked fit, that was enough. Most people didn't even have that, right? Keep in mind I was young and female and the dialogue I had been programed with was all about the external. It was all about looking good and nothing to do with feeling well. Clearly I had a lot of work to do.

Fast forward to having my second son, Sam. I was 32 and the nodules on my thyroid had multiplied to a total of nine masses. One was actually bigger than my thyroid itself and my last thyroid panel showed my TSH at less than .0001. Let's just say that's really not what you want. Your endocrine system kind of regulates everything and if your thyroid burns out of hormone your entire system eventually shuts down. I had started having symptomatic *stuff* that included mild tremors, more frequent panic attacks, extreme fatigue, and bouts of mild depression. I was having what they call mini thyroid *storms*. I was scared for myself and I was even more scared for my kids. If I couldn't figure out what was going on with me how was I going to protect, teach, and raise my children to be healthy? Was I even going to be around for them?

So, I put my momma warrior pants on and began to invoke my own inner unicorn and thought if this were happening to one of my kids what would I do? I needed to do that for myself.

I eventually had my thyroid removed. For me, it was the right choice at the time. At the rate it was going it wasn't going to last my lifetime and I basically shortcut the step of letting it burn out. I embarked on a lifetime of chemical meds to replace my little butterfly organ and marched towards writing my own food reset. I knew my major issues were food related. I never let anyone convince me otherwise. Though I had yet to truly discover my inner unicorn, I was unbelievably stubborn when it came to my feelings, my intuition. I still am … and forever will be. Unrelenting commitment to my intuition has saved my life more than once.

Intuition — the mark of a unicorn. Looking back, I had been a unicorn all the time (you are too) I just hadn't owned it, named it, or identified it. I didn't know I could carry fistfulls of glitter, even in the darkest of days. I never let anyone talk me out of what I knew to be *true* about my body, even when it made zero practical sense. Listening to the general consensus would have negated my personal intuition. It would have gone against what my soul knew was the correct path for healing. I have always believed you are what you eat and that your gut instincts are always right.

I believed, as I still do, that food is fuel — beautifully nourishing and absolutely healing. I had always eaten *healthy* but it wasn't working for me. I devoured articles and books on food sensitivity, intolerance, leaky gut, celiac, and thyroid dysfunction. I relentlessly searched symptoms in an effort to connect pieces and chatted with my endocrinologist about my suspicions. I took blood tests, skin tests, elimination diets, and cleanses. In the midst of it all, I cracked my own code and saw very clearly how others could figure out how to *balance* their own systems. I became my own wellness detective. My personal wellness doula.

I discovered that certain things absolutely didn't work for me no matter how many articles or practitioners said they were "packed with nutrients" and "good" for your best health.

My first step was to remove gluten. Although I had always tested negative for gluten sensitivity … and still do … I removed it from my diet and immediately (within four days) had a solid bowel movement. Too much information perhaps, I know, but bowel movements are one of the clearest markers of your internal health. They are a beautifully simple reality check. I thought "AHA! This is it! I ditch gluten and the world is my oyster! I AM A UNICORN!"

Not quite.

I eliminated gluten and continued to eat things that were supposedly healing and healthy but things just didn't *fix* and then — because the universe, as blessed and glittering as it is, can have a nasty sense of humor in the name of teaching us our lessons in this physical life — I went through a time period where things got worse.

I went back to the drawing board. I did more reading, more experimenting. I knew gluten was out, but I was also becoming suspicious of nuts, nightshades, and a myriad of other foods and ingredients. I kept thinking perhaps EVERYTHING was cross-contaminated with gluten. But no, I was not responding to many other things, just nuts, seeds, nightshades, any grain-fed animal, "natural flavorings," "artificial flavors," legumes, and all grains, plus casein. I researched every possible gut irritant and thoughtfully and methodically took them all out. I kept in foods that I had researched and found to be healing, non-irritating to the digestive tract, and easy to absorb nutritionally. I also researched how to get the most nutrients out of your foods, cooking methods, cooked vs. raw, and created a balanced map that had me feeling better than I EVER thought possible.

The research I did ended up becoming the food Reset. My Reset is included in the back of this handbook … with some additional recommendations for Unicorns, specifically because, feeding a unicorn is an incredibly important step in invoking your unicorn power. Within 21 days of doing my first, personal Reset I had identified more foods that were triggers for my sensitive belly than I had in my entire lifetime! I felt empowered, vibrant, rested, and above all armed with a road map for myself. I felt magical. I cracked my own food code! It was what I needed, not what anyone else said it should be. the Reset custom built my nutritional road map from my own body! I felt mythic when I ate the foods that I know work for me. I still do! I live and abide by my personal Reset findings and still allow them to evolve, but I always honor the conversation with my body — don't worry, we'll get to all the goods on this later in the handbook.

Becoming a unicorn is about becoming your most vibrant, balanced, and healthy self and working with your own needs and responses. Learning what works and what doesn't work for your body, mind, and spirit regardless of what any expert (yup, mocking myself here), doctor, therapist, spiritual guru, motivational speaker, teacher, specialist, nutritionist, or dietician says.

I believe each unicorn needs something different in order to shine their brightest. You can *crack your own code* with the food Reset in a short time — minus a ton of pricey testing — which I've done and you should do if you think you have genuine health issues triggered by food and have insurance to cover it, but those don't always give you functional answers or real life help. ALL of my testing came back negative for years. I never did and still do not have any food allergies. I have however, been diagnosed by my general practitioner and endocrinologist with Celiac based on my reactions to gluten.

We've all gotten a bit too wrapped up and dependent on the mechanical, analytical testing. Tests continue to come back normal … and yet you are still symptomatic and feel awful.

Tests are a necessary step and a benchmark but they aren't the entire full truth or the definitive answer.

If you feel terrible,you feel terrible. How you feel is real and regardless of what the tests say you need tangible ways to make your body and self better.

Thanks to the Food Reset I know what sets my system off. I'm not perfect and I still trip up, but I am healthier than I've ever been and am able to fully embrace my unicorn spirit! I'm not crazy fatigued anymore. I don't have to take a nap every afternoon with my boys simply to make it to dinner time. I no longer have panic attacks or extreme anxiety. I feel safe in my body and generally happy, capable, and vibrant in the world. Above all I am capable of caring, teaching, and raising my children and my community of clients, and members to listen to their systems; body, mind, and spirit to create the highest health for themselves.

Our wellness is not just about our vanity. It's about our longevity and quality of life. Teaching is my way of loving. It's what I have to give and my way of showing up in the world. I'm here to give as many people as possible a path to a calm, balanced, healthy experience in their body. I want to throw a giant hot pink bubble of love around each of you and shout "YOU ARE A UNICORN! I LOVE YOU! GO BE

AMAZING! You just need a few practices to be MAGICAL!"

This handbook and my online studio (www.matandkitchen.com — more on this later) are what I wished for when I was going through my unicorn evolution. Wellness should be about being of use and service to the world and the people we care about. Accessible, efficient, clear but deep, full of love, intellect, and intuition.

There are so many things in life to experience and I'll be damned if I or any of you are going to miss out on any of it because we haven't learned to honor ourselves and our systems and our loves above all else.

We all know we *should* address our health and spiritual connection but what we don't always know is how or our why's.

My Why's

My *Why's* on becoming my own unicorn are named Milo, Sam, Mateo, Marco and every client that has ever connected with me. My children husband and step-son are more gorgeous and powerful teachers than I ever could have imagined and I want to be the most I can be, for them. I wake up every morning trying to show up better for them. I'm not always successful … but the intent is there. Like a morning mantra or prayer, each day I try, I aim for the better, for them and for me.

My other *Whys* are my clients, members, subscribers, and community. I genuinely want to sprinkle fistfulls of glitter all over the people I connect with. I want to spread unicorn magic like oxygen to help as many people as I possibly can feel amazing! IT'S POSSIBLE! UNICORN MAGIC IS REAL!

But you have to believe. I'm here to make you a believer.

How to be a Unicorn

The *How* is all about tending to ourselves with respect through the self-care techniques I'll teach in this handbook to balance your body on both the physical and energetic levels with equal length, strength, and mobility without over-taxing or burning out your system. Balance in all things brings results. Unicorn balance is created with equal strength and flexibility, activity and rest, clean food and hydration, meditation and the magic of spiritual rituals.

How I Became a Unicorn

I launched a subscription-based lifestyle website in February 2013. I had gone from full-time working momma in the fitness industry teaching, training, managing a group fitness program, and Regional Pilates Manager to part-time working momma training clients via Skype and traveling to teach workshops to full-time stay-at-home-momma, to I-want-to-work-and-have-more-to-give-to-the-world-but-don't-want-to-be-away-from-my-boys-very-much momma.

Enter my incredibly supportive, brilliant, and creative husband. After we went rounds and rounds about what I would do next work-wise he suggested we build an online offering. He'd watched me teach six to eight hours a day, five days a week for years and knew content was not an issue. He knew that I was a worker bee and performer all rolled into one and he just kept championing an online subscription-based offering.

Please keep in mind this was over five years ago now and NO ONE was doing online fitness on their own. It was all big companies shifting from DVD production to online plug and play offerings. Online fitness wasn't personal. It wasn't boutique and you never knew the quality of the trainer you were getting.

It was a complete leap of faith to build our own platform that was connected and caring and real, with workouts in real time, macro- and micro-cycled on the back end and new every three days.

•

It was an offering just as if you walked into a multi-level class (it still is … it's alive and well and thriving!) … it was just online.

I had never shot video on my own before, never edited, color corrected, exported, or uploaded. It was all a learning curve. My perfectionist nature was terrified. I thought an online offering had to be big bucks with a massive production team.

This was another unicorn transformation. I had to let go of the perfectionism and work with what we had. I proceeded with the affirmation *I am enough. Just as I am.* If I waited to be perfect … well … I'd have never become a unicorn and I certainly never would have launched an online subscription-based website. If I had stayed in the comfort of my perfectionism I never would have put a single video up.

My husband and I created PimpYourMat.com in February 2013. Two years later it transitioned to www.matandkitchen.com. It grew from a simple offering of 30-minute mat-based workouts to over 300 dairy- and gluten-free recipes, my 41-Day Food Reset, a newsletter, 30 Days to Better online courses, multiple private Facebook groups for members and access to me as your actual coach and trainer to go to for modifications, adjustments, motivation, and support.

UnicorWellness.Studio solved our family's needs and the needs of every other busy person who is trying to stay or get balanced and fit in a tech-savvy, time-efficient, budget-honoring, intelligent way.

We created my online studio as a creative way for me to spend more time with our boys but I also wanted to embark on this adventure because I wanted to try and make a dent in the frustrating and disempowering offerings of the fitness industry. Especially for women.

We launched an online offering with a unique voice to try and break through the noise of fitness and make a genuine impact on wellness. Launching my online offering was about calling bullshit on the ads, marketing and methods of the fitness industry. I felt called to preach and teach the truth of personal evolution and genuine wellness results that last a lifetime rather than just 30, 60 or 90 days.

Getting fit and healthy is all about getting real, simple, and honest and no one was even coming close to teaching that.

Not to say *no one* teaches the real goods. Those intelligent, educated, loving teachers and coaches are out there. Sadly, they just aren't the loudest or the most well known.

Most people genuinely think fitness and wellness are difficult, time-consuming, costly, and down right confusing, so why bother? People think getting healthy is hard. Or that it's an endless catch-22 or that it's only maintainable for 30-, 60-, or 90-days at a time.

I've spent my entire adult career in the fitness industry, many of those years with a dirty little secret — that I was physically fit and lean but internally a health mess.

I became a wellness unicorn to dispel as many of the false paradigms and myths PR and marketing have fed us and to make the process of becoming your most magical self accessible, efficient, and fun.

I became a wellness unicorn to teach the differences between fitness and wellness and to be the bridge from fitness to wellness.

I, and my online wellness center, take a kind and consistent approach to balancing a body. I teach you how to listen and connect with your own system without it getting sleepy or lame. Unicorn Wellness has a thriving community of members worldwide who support and motivate each other along their wellness journeys. Basically my husband and I built a virtual brick and mortar studio *online*. Real people, real stories, real connections, and real results.

I know the majority of my members by name, their stories, their wins, and their fails. I'm in it with them. Every day online. I want to be an advocate for all those who feel lost along their wellness way and for others to know they don't have to be at the mercy of their bodies. I want you to know can be fit and well without beating yourself up.

I'm grateful that my journey is now helping so many others fast-track their wellness. The most important lesson I've learned in my journey with IBS, Celiac, and a thyroidectomy is that you don't need major medical issues to warrant wanting to feel better. Again, I'm blown away by how many people just simply don't feel good. It makes me sad. Life is meant to be seized, lived, and enjoyed, and you need energy and clarity of mind for that. You need a happy, joyful, well-balanced body. In other words, you need to be a unicorn.

I'll guide you to discover/realize that your life is full of infinite possibilities. I'll teach you to be a unicorn via body, mind, and spirit.

My Unicorn Evolutions

I ultimately became a unicorn many times over the years and intend to continue to do so for the rest of my life, but my true transformation has come in three pieces:

First, I became a unicorn in my physical body on the mat after we launched my first online fitness offering. I quit doing all the other crazy workouts and all the "new" fitness trends every year and finally only did my own workouts — the ones I wrote. My second transformation was in the kitchen when I wrote my 41-Day Food Reset and I cracked my own food code — the code that I had struggled to find answers to for 12 years. This one was fascinating because the unicorn invocation through food happened more deeply in my mind and emotions than in my physical body — and the body transformation was powerful. My third major unicorn transition manifested a few years later when I anchored into my spiritual rituals of tarot and daily meditation. This was the most magical and the piece that connected and amplified everything else.

'Unicorn' but Not in the Good Way …

In 2015 my family I moved from Brooklyn, NY back to Austin, TX. I say back, because we had lived there before. We'd done the bounce from LA, Austin, back to LA, to NY then back to Austin and yes, if you follow me on social media … you'll know we are currently back in Brooklyn … oh how Paulo Coelho's *The Alchemist* rings true in our lives. We chose to go back to Austin. At that time I thought I wanted to buy a forever house with a backyard for my boys and to have all our children in one place. The reality was, we were transitioning the online studio to our primary income and I was terrified to live in New York. I was scared it wouldn't last and New York's cost of living felt daunting at the time. I never actually voiced this (red flag on the unicorn front … not listening to

your inside voice, your gut, your instinct …
NEVER goes well. In fact, it's the exact
recipe for a "learning opportunity." We all
know that term is code for difficult times
and trouble, yes?). But I felt it. I was scared
to raise two (three including my step-son)
kiddos on the income of what began as a
side project.

I never thought, when we launched Pimp
Your Mat, which turned into Mat & Kitchen,
and is now UnicorWellness.Studio…….
that we'd ever live off of it. I had no vision
originally. No business plan. Zero intention
of this being our primary source of income.

My husband and I talked about embracing
the fact we had no tethers. No reason to
stay in New York, every opportunity to live
a #lifebydesign and do whatever, wherever
we wanted. Clearly we were gypsies in a
past life. We have gypsy souls. We allowed
our conversations to take us in the

direction that security was better in Austin and *if* something ever went wrong with the business we'd be *safer* in Austin. Please note the avid use of italics in this section … more red flags from the universe.

This period of time of planning our move to Austin was a funny and sneaky one. We were excited, we were talking through everything and it all sounded like excellent adulting … and really, really *safe*.

Unicorns, please note, that the feelings and use of words like *safe* or *adult* are also red flags to your ultimate unicorn nature. These are excuses and blockades to your unique greatness. *Safe* and *Adult* tend to adopt an idea of "normal" that does nothing but prevent us from our personal best and flat out give the universe permission to school us on what is real.

The words safe and adult cut you off from the magic of your inner child and your inner unicorn in one giant swoop. They instill fear.

Safe and adult disconnect you from your internal personal compass. It's the stuff that stops you from doing …right before you're about to have the most amazing breakthrough.

I felt, in my gut, that it wasn't the right thing to do. That it wasn't the right move to head back to Austin but I continued to have conversations and I agreed to move. I allowed the analytical pros to outweigh the intuitive cons. I never voiced my actual fears to my husband; I rode the wave that took us back to Austin.

I don't want to take up this entire book with this particular story. But it is a poignant one. It's the time that allowed me to learn that my *feels* are real. My often inexplicable feelings, intuition, and gut instincts have always turned out to be truer than my analytical lists with supporting evidence, and that when I don't voice them … there's bound to be a mess to clean up.

When we arrived in Austin we had the best of intentions. We found a house in the "perfect" neighborhood — within walking distance of schools for both the boys and a studio space for filming workouts. Then our moving truck arrived. And I kid you not, nearly everything was shattered. Up to this point we had moved as a family a total of six times. Never had we had out things so ruined. The moving company literally threw our things in boxes and everything was destroyed. If this sign wasn't a clear enough sign, the house ended up having critters in the walls (racoons and yes, even a rat) and to top it off, the house was haunted. Momma handled that one with three "clearings" but they were stubborn and there were many a sleepless or interrupted sleep night in our two and a half years there. My oldest son was bullied at school and, well, in general … it wasn't anywhere near idyllic, easier or safe. Brooklyn was a dream in comparison … seven-month winters and all.

At every turn in Austin we tried. I can say this absolutely. We just kept handling each "lesson" that showed up. Friends I had had before acted super weird to me, didn't want to connect or hang out, I was called an "uptight-East Coaster" because I made my oldest kid do his homework before a playdate, I was constantly called out for the way our family ate (we abide by our food codes) in highly judgmental and derogatory ways. I went to every school function and networking event that I could find and was continually passive aggressively insulted or blown off. I'd set up meetings with businesses we wanted to partner with and continually get this particular *look* I'd not experienced before. And please keep in mind I was born and raised in the South. I'm from Oklahoma and my mother absolutely doesn't believe you're dressed unless you have lipstick on, and no, gloss doesn't count.

I'd come home from a meeting with someone and Mateo would take one look at me and say, "Did it happen again?" and I'd say yes and then try to explain the experience. Until one day after yet another strange meeting, I blurted out, "They just keep looking at me like I've got something sticking out of my head … like I'm a unicorn … but not the good kind … like I'm too driven, too hungry … just too *something*." And I'll tell you in all my time in Los Angeles and New York I've never had meetings like these where people would actually insult your business but still want access to your community with zero exchange or give on their part. In LA and New York people are keenly aware of six degrees of separation and they make an art of gracefully getting out of things or passing on projects that still leaves the relationship intact … juuuuuust in case further down the road your paths cross and you want to work together. Austin just kept throwing out whammies.

I had never identified with unicorns before. Sure, I always liked to sparkle and shine. I owned My Little Ponies as a kid. I always believed in serendipity, coincidence, the law of attraction, miracles, and magic. But I wasn't much for unicorns before this. It was simply the only way I could explain the look people gave me. The feeling of being the ultimate outsider. Like they'd never seen anything like me before and they had no idea what to do with me. They were attracted to me but appalled at the same time. At the time it hurt my feelings. At the time it made me feel like I was 12 and had changed schools and didn't have anyone to sit with at lunch. It poked on every raw place of feeling unwanted, unworthy and not belonging I had — and man, did I have a lot of those places.

My Austin experience made me feel incredibly lonely, like I was doing all the wrong things and making wrong choices. I started to anchor into this idea of a unicorn and went to work on learning the symbolism and historical reference point for them. I began to embrace this square peg round hole experience and started to own my inner unicorn and went about invoking it. On my terms. With a positive flip of the script.

I went from wounded and hurt to … you're damn straight you're looking at a unicorn … you want to be a part of this magic or not? Not? Okay, please step aside. I've got glitter to throw and light to shine and you're blocking the path.

I was lonely in Austin. And please know, I love Austin. I have nothing against it. It's a lovely place. This particular experience had everything to do with my personal lessons, for which I am forever grateful for because otherwise, I wouldn't be teaching you how to embrace your personal unicorn vibes and shine bright as you possibly can in the world. I had my work and my family but I was feeling incredibly empty and isolated in the realm of community and spirit. As I navigated my feelings with my intuitive feels I kept getting the feeling I needed to pull out the deck of tarot cards I'd owned since I was 16 and finally make a diligent, consistent practice of my meditation rather than the spotty hobby streaks I'd lived with for over 20 years.

For all intents and purposes, my third unicorn transformation was a full-fledged awakening. The outside world was testing me. I could no longer simply feel fulfilled with the getting and the doing — I needed something more, bigger, and much more magical in my life. I needed to know how to balance and navigate my intuition, how to get those things to work for me and my family rather than feeling as if we were actively working against them. I needed a time and space to empty out the negative vibes and fill up on the positive highs that were all offered in meditation and in the cards.

After about a year of the *bad unicorn* experiences I tinkered with my tarot cards every Sunday. Like going to church. I'd wait till everyone was in bed because I just couldn't deal with anymore inquiry or conversation on *me* (though my family has been unbelievably supportive in my unicorn transformation). I needed the time to just be mine for a bit in the beginning. Without the eyes, the suggestions or the conversation. I set a ritual day and time and simply stayed consistent. I was constantly frustrated and confused for quite a while but I kept shuffling, pulling, and reading the cards.

And I meditated. I set up an altar I loved. FIlled it with crystals and candles and incense, and truly felt supported every time I sat in front of it. I didn't make any *have to*'s on this one. I just went to sit. I'd listen to music, binaural beats, guided, chanting … I'd do it in silence, I'd ask questions or I wouldn't, I'd hold a crystal or not, I'd lie down or I'd sit. I just showed up and explored and appreciated the quiet. I realized it was working its magic by creating calm and space, more joy and less caring of what others thought. Fast forward three years, it's a daily practice …

every day … sometimes twice a day if I'm called.

Do I miss one now and then? Sure. I do it thoughtfully and I honor that life is busy and complicated. I know that on days I don't meditate, I'm still a child of God and supported by the universe. There is no perfect, in anything. There is integrity, consistency and practice. These rest is noise that diverts the process and progress.

Through meditation I began to feel anchored and calm, more focused, lighter. … Yup, I began to feel all the things you read about feeling after you have a meditation practice. It's all true. And there's no way to impart that until you try. There's research, there is history, there are stories, there's practice — and then there's the reality of experience.

We think that meditation will be like popping an aspirin and in 20 minutes the joy and calm, clarity and focus just flip to the on position. When in reality the process is slow and sneaky. It's an undercurrent that swells up to lighten the dark, heavy layers of life.

My final unicorn transformation happened in spirit. Talk about the need to *lean in* and take a seat at the table. I pulled up my chair to the spiritual table and now refuse to leave. I finally embraced the practices I had embarked on at 16. The books, the cards, the meditation, chakras, energies, crystals … all of it. I re-experienced all the habits and tactics my religious southern mother told me were "of the dark" or "of the devil" and weren't allowed in her house … and I finally felt like I was home.

The strangely systematic comfort of the tarot ordered my thoughts, intuition, and feels. They allowed me to articulate the things I *knew* (clairvoyance) but couldn't explain and allowed me to finally feel supported, loving, and useful to others in a way nothing ever had before.

The magic of meditation and the tarot crafted an anchor for this unicorn in the most delicious way. It was also the most ironic journey … that began when I was 16 but took me 20 years to return to. It was my final piece of the triad. Mind, body, and spirit — fully present in this physical life by getting lost in the stars. Like having all of my limbs on one body again I began to prance with my unicorn horn rather than stumble over my magic. I had a place to come to and lay out all the confusion and feels, a place to know it's all okay, every part of our life experience, evolution, and journey to *better*.

What I Teach

I continue to practice a blend of western and alternative medicines, self-care, intelligent and balanced workouts, hydration, and real food to keep me showing up in the world as a unicorn. Most trainers, magazines, marketing, and PR unfortunately are still functioning from a fear factor: telling the world to beat a body up rather than educate and empower. I teach empowerment. I teach the invocation of healing. When you head down the path of becoming a unicorn you aim at the better, nothing more and nothing less.

I teach a bridge of fitness and spirituality that leads straight to wellness. Fitness and wellness are two different things but they can sew together in the most beautiful of ways to create strength, goodness, and joy from the inside out. It's a paradigm shift to think that if we actually back off a bit, we'll get better results. A unicorn learns that by doing less you actually get more.

Sparkle and Shine Never Go Out of Style

Being a unicorn is about awareness and connection. I keep it simple and teach life tactics to get more out of doing less because you're working smarter, not harder, in harmony with how a body actually functions.

Remember, there really aren't any new ideas, there are however new ways to communicate and share them. Everyone needs a teacher and there's a teacher out there for everyone. I hope to be yours but you'll need to trust me. Because the goods of getting to personal unicorn status aren't earth shattering, in fact, you may find them utterly banal. Simplicity and consistency are pure magic. There are answers in the silence and there is magic in you. These steps on how to be a unicorn are so simple you may laugh. Just realize, when you laugh, not only do you burn 10 calories, you raise your vibration, you invoke your inner child, the true essence of a unicorn, the delight and joy of a pure spirit. So, laugh it up, then get into the assignments to do the simple steps to be a unicorn! Because as they say, life will pass regardless, do you want to do it with sparkle and shine or do you want to remain in the fear and struggle? The choice is always yours.

Unicorn Reality

I've written a handbook because the truth is, you don't need a 350-page book to get you to your most magical. You need real, tangible, gimmick-free, actionable techniques that have a proven track record. You need habits you can start NOW, not plan to implement in the weeks after you've (maybe) finished the book. I'm always looking at ways to make things more intelligent and more efficient. Life is full and busy, you need your self evolution to be well balanced, straightforward, and simple.

More is not better. More often keeps you stuck in your past stories of *trying* and never succeeding or evolving. Less *is* the new more. Take this handbook and invoke your inner unicorn. No need to waste time or indulge in unnecessary pages.

Tools for Unicorn Transformation

If you want to take your unicorn transformation to the next level, in addition to this handbook you'll eventually want a membership to my website in order to be able to workout with me #onthemat. (Or at least I hope you do!) The physical body must be addressed for full unicorn invocation. To support and facilitate this I created a cost- and schedule-efficient, accessible offering online.

You can join me in my online studio for 30 minute mat-based workouts, brand new every three days, macro- and micro-cycled on the back end in perpetuity for you in true personal training form (pilates and yoga based) at www.matandkitchen.com. You'll also have access to over 300 gluten- and dairy-free recipes, the condensed PDF version of my 41 Day Food Reset (but you've got the expanded version in this handbook … YAY for bonuses!), access to three private Facebook groups, my monthly newsletter and the current 30 Days to Better online courses, and me.

You also have access to my monthly, new and full moon tarot readings, plus a monthly guided meditation to support the exploration of your soul. These videos are a gift to use and share on your unicorn path. Dig deep, be informed and armed with the transiting energies each month so you're never caught by surprise on your path forward, but instead bolstered, knowledgeable and as many steps ahead of the curve as you can be because you go beyond this earthly experience and navigate with a divine GPS.

30 Days to Be a Unicorn

I wrote this handbook to be implemented within 30 days. One month to your personal magic. The techniques and tactics are broken down in a week-by-week format. You'll have one practical or magical tactic to focus on each week.

Can you read ahead? Yes! Of course, enthusiasm is always rewarded!

Can you implement the practices 'out of order'? Sure, Week #4 could easily and happily be Week #1 but you do need to use all the offerings in tandem to truly achieve unicorn status.

That being said, layer in what you can when you can. Your path is yours, your schedule is yours, don't create excuses that prevent you from starting or doing at least some of these practices. My teaching motto is *Better is Better.* Doing something towards your sparkle and shine is exponentially better than doing nothing. Ditch the guilt the *shoulds* and the idea of perfection. It doesn't exist. Better exists. Healing exists. Unicorns exist.

To become a unicorn you will work through four weeks via this handbook. Simply start reading.

Your four weeks of unicorn training are broken down as follows:

Week 1 - Workouts & Hydration
Week 2 - Fuel & How to Feed a Unicorn (My 41-Day Food Reset)
Week 3 - Self Care
Week 4 - Spiritual Ritual

My hope is to create a loving, clear, concise experience that lives with you outside of these pages. I don't just write this handbook then leave you. I'm online every day, in real time, week-to-week to continue to support, motivate, and help you practice your personal unicorn evolution.

You can read this handbook and walk away … or you can read it then hop online and cultivate your sparkle and shine with me by your side every day. You can have the support of the Unicorn Wellness community via social media … or not. You're not alone — if you don't want to be.

This is the true beauty and potential of the internet, to have a real, genuine, personal, boutique online studio experience. I teach in real time with real people in the mix with you … if you want it.

Unicorn Transformation Begins!

WEEK ONE

In week one you'll embark on a fitness and wellness education that will change the way you look at *results* in your health and wellness.

ASSIGNMENT 1: WORKOUTS

To fully experience your unicorn transformation you'll want to become a member in my online studio —

www.matandkitchen.com. Can you still read this handbook and implement the steps? Yes! Of course. Will the movement portion make as much sense or be as connected if you're not working out with me? Not really.

But it's ok! Everything in divine time, not on my time. If it's not time for you to hop into my online studio … simply read the sections and implement them as best you can. If you do nothing but read it, it's expanding your perspective and education on connected and aware workouts.

If it is divine timing for you to train with me simply head over to www.unicornwellnessstudio.com and *sign-up with promo code **UNICORN** to zero out your cart for 30 days free on the site. You'll also get a 30-day rewind so you can use all of the workouts posted in the previous month to begin your membership.

This is a $64 value for free 'cause unicorns spread love and resources when and where they can! You can cancel at anytime, it's two button clicks from your account on the site and no catch- 22.

Membership to my studio gives you access to a full circle wellness center at the tip of your fingers. UnicorWellness.Studio is truly a wellness home and knowing that there is no such thing as coincidence … it's most likely yours because you've picked up this handbook.

*your account will automatically rollover to a paid account on day 31 if you do not cancel within 24 hours prior. The paid account is $32 a month.

I macro- and micro-cycle all of your workouts in perpetuity. If you are #onthemat with me you are getting true personal training that optimizes your progress in strength, mobility, flexibility, healing, and injury prevention. Just press play to train with me. You can hop into the flow at any time.

Unicornwellnessstudio.com workouts are for all fitness levels. Every workout is crafted as if you walked into a mixed level class in a brick and mortar studio. Simply meet yourself #onthemat each time and do as much as you can by following my cuing … not by trying to do exactly what I do. Everybody is coming to their wellness journey from a unique place. We honor that #onthemat.

You NEVER need to do anything but log in to your account and do the workout of the day. The 'Just Press Play' method reaps the best results and allows me to do my job as your personal trainer. There's no need to create chaos and confusion. If you knew how to program your workouts for best results you wouldn't need me. Allow yourself to let relax and enjoy and just do.

Every 30-minute workout video is live on the site as the V.O.D. — the video of the day — for three days each. Then is stashed in your personal account to go back to at any time if necessary.

Day 1 of the workout is to get acquainted with it. Day 2 of the workout allows you to go deeper in the work. Day 3 of the workout allows you to have some mastery over that series.

Then we transition to a new workout for muscle and brain variation — no boredom, no autopilot — true periodization in your movement for actual results in your fitness and wellness.

One week of every month is a full stretch week for constructive rest, at the new moon.
Two weeks of the month are medium effort workouts.
One week of every month is harder than the rest.

Every other workout on the site uses a prop. You do not need to buy all the props at once, I rotate through them over time. If you'd like to see them or purchase what you don't have, you can find my favorites at the Props link at the bottom of the page at www.tandygutierrez.com here. If you don't have the current prop you can do the workout prior or try the Video of the Day without the prop.

As a member of UnicorWellness.Studio you'll receive my monthly newsletter, which arrives with the new moon every month. I share the monthly cosmic and seasonal energy we are working with, questions to work with to improve your personal magic inside and out, links to my free monthly guided meditation and tarot readings, plus specific healing crystal and essential oil recommendations particular to each month so you have everything you need to balance your mind, body and spirit in real time.

The current collective astrology + lunar cycles of each month are taken into account and tended to in your 30 minute workouts to balance a body energetically as well as physically.

Regardless of how you choose to workout, pick a realistic number of workouts to commit to for the next 30 days. Don't pick how many times you *think* you should do.

Pick what your life allows. Unicorns are built on consistency, intellect and hope, we don't hold on to our stories of *trying* or flat out failure. Unicorns do not make excuses. We make things happen. We balance the earthly physical issues with a magical connection to the divine. We throw some glitter on the mess of reality and transform it into sparkle and shine.

1. Create a schedule that allows you to be consistent. Answer the following: What times and what days am I going to get #onthemat with Tandy? Where will I do my workouts? How many workouts can I actually get done in my week versus how many I *want* to do?

2. Two workouts are the minimum recommendation to instigate healing and empowered balance. The sweet spot is four to six times a week #onthemat with me for the four weeks of your unicorn transformation. Success comes from consistency.

Sparkle and Shine by Design … Not by Default

Your unicorn workouts with me each week will consist of 30-minute mat-based workouts rooted in pilates but flavored with yoga, functional movement, and basic resistance training designed to heal a body. unicornwellnessstudio.com workouts create equal strength, mobility, and flexibility in your physical body while also clearing stuck energies that block your capacity to manifest and evolve for the better.

All of my workouts are appropriate for all fitness levels. That being said, the goal is for you to start a conversation with your body every time you get #onthemat. Meet yourself #onthemat.

I don't teach a specific *beginner, intermediate,* or *advanced* series because after 20+ years of teaching and training, I know that bodies don't really work that way. Bodies are a mixture of levels and you'll surprise yourself as to what you're capable of doing without the false concepts or *label* of where you should or want to be. This speaks just as loudly to those of us that think we are *advanced* as it does to those that are just beginning. Advanced students can be the worst of the bunch (I get to say this because I was totally one of these people and can still be, because I'm human along with my unicorn-ness) because we can power and plow through tricks without bringing true alignment, connection, or awareness to the work.

I teach a multi-level class in every video, because it's important to remain open, to not set limits or expectations (low or high), and to simply come to the mat, listen, approach what you can, and leave what isn't a fit yet, in an intelligent and supportive way. I offer distinctive cuing that guides you to where your body can take you, that day. There are always options for different bodies and body types.

In my teaching experience this puts everyone on as even a playing field as possible, allowing for progress, healing, and evolution … faster, efficiently and safely. This is where #lessisthenewmore comes in. Like I said earlier, you'll need to trust me. You'll be shocked at how time #onthemat with me is so general and yet so personal. It's part of the unicorn magic. You'll just have to experience it to understand it.

My workouts are excellent for small spaces, travel, and packed schedules. You can do them anywhere you have a wifi connection. On your smartphone, tablet, laptop, or desktop. And I prefer you to come with zero experience or expectations. Be open. The way you approach your physical body #onthemat is often how we approach life. Work #onthemat offers unlimited learning and positive evolution of ourselves to simply be in the moment, meeting ourselves on the mat, with what our bodies are capable of doing that day, in that moment that we can carry directly #offthemat.

These workouts are not super sweaty (you don't always need to shower afterwards). If you know you are particularly tight you may want to have a set of yoga blocks and a yoga strap handy to best support your body.

These workouts are also super suited to those with chronic issues or injuries. Being on the mat with me can support your body to heal in a way few, if anything else, can.

What to Expect When You Work Out with Me

Results may come slower and much sneakier with UnicorWellness.Studio workouts but the knowledge you gain from them will last a lifetime because my workouts address your bone and muscle structure via proper alignment and hormone balance. UnicorWellness.Studio workouts guide you back into proper anatomical alignment with attention to your bones and how they stack. This allows your muscles, ligaments, and tendons to lie and connect in the way they are meant to. Working out with me is like taking all the wiring behind your TV and instead of leaving it in a jumbled, tangled mess, it's sorted out in neat lines and labeled with color coded tags. Proper alignment brings faster results. Working out with me heals injuries and prevents future ones. Working out with UnicorWellness.Studio creates core strength that is unparalleled. You will experience intelligent, calm and kind body work #onthemat with me.

Quality over Quantity

I macro- and micro-cycle your workouts behind the scenes. For all the fitness geeks out there this will mean something. For the non-fitness geeks it simply means I'm taking care of your strength, flexibility, rest, recovery, balanced range and planes of motion to create a balanced, uninjured body that will get stronger and deliver results … just as any good personal trainer does.

I don't randomly shoot workouts. There is a method to the unicorn madness to keep you continually making progress. Working out with me is personal training, like you walked into a small group mixed-level class with me weekly. If you are ever confused or need to ask a question, you can, via social media.

In contrast, DVDs are the same workout over and over. They are static and when you workout with them you quickly learn exactly how long it takes, what's coming next and how much energy to save for it, as well as skipping or zoning out during the parts you don't like.

Other online options may seem more "studio-esque" but they're nothing more than a plug and play. Allowing unending options for you to pick, stress, and fret over. I'm telling you right now this might be worse than a DVD.

Randomly picking a workout doesn't work. A workout or dedicated movement practice shouldn't be random. When you, as a consumer and student get to pick your workouts you're literally adding insult to injury. You pick what you think you need.

You pick what you want. Not what your body needs or requires for optimal health and fitness. You'll pick things that create or drive home imbalances. You'll pick what you like, and what you like is what you're good and strong at, leaving the weak parts farther and farther behind.

A body is a beautiful connected system and needs someone who understands how it works to tend to it's journey and progress. That's what experts are for. You may be in an expert in something, you want people to come to you to allow your gifts to shine … not everyone is an expert in fitness and wellness and shouldn't be in the driver's seat for periodization and exercise choices.

Your workouts, fitness, or movement should be enjoyable but be clear, it's not entertainment. It's not like picking a show to watch. There is a purpose and a method to getting healthy results and that process should reflect the purpose and results you are working towards.

This is a huge reason most people don't get results even for all their effort. They don't know what they're doing with their overall movement.There is an art and intelligence to mapping movements.

I create variation every three days on UnicorWellness.Studio to keep your brain and body progressing and not zoning out. It generates enough repetition to create mastery over time, and enough variation to keep your brain and body constantly engaged, ever evolving, and always progressing towards a more magical you.

30 Minutes is Enough to Make Magic

It works. I teach you to work on the mat in harmony with your body, not against it, so you get more results for life — not just for 30, 60, or 90 days. Forget what you think you know about fitness. I can get you more by doing less. Thirty-minute workouts allow for life.

I realize body wellness is my passion. I love the process and the topic, but you may not want to consume your life with the ins and outs of taking care of your physical body. That's okay! You don't need to! Thirty minutes is enough to get results, while leaving you plenty of time for everything else you have and want to do. Keeping workouts to 30 minutes also prevents your body from firing stress hormones, which are a major issue for those of us with autoimmune issues, but also for nearly everyone over the age of 35 or post natal (doesn't matter when the *post* was) or if you have a menstrual cycle or are navigating the perimenopausal or postmenopausal journey.

As adults, male or female, our bodies are typically battling hormone imbalance from the years of workouts that blasted our adrenal glands, chemicals in our foods, cleaning products, the air we breathe, or simply the shift of stages in life. Body wellness is actually a result of hormone balance, so when you keep to the 30 minute marker of working out you avoid firing the stress hormones that can thwart progress. Hence, more is not better, especially when it comes to a workout. This is a larger conversation we'll save for another time and another book, but trust me, it's real. This is one of the two main reasons I finally started to heal and thrive with my autoimmune diseases. I quit doing what everyone thought was *optimal* for *fitness* and started listening to my system and researching what I was experiencing and connecting the dots. Thirty minutes works. That's really all you need to know.

What About Cardio?

When it comes to frequently asked questions this ranks at the tippy top. Some of you will rejoice with what I'm going to say and others, well … you'll pull that side-eye out real fast. When it comes to well-rounded wellness you're going to need a bit of cardio. For your heart. Because, let's all get clear, that's what cardio is really for. The cardiac muscle. Cardio is for your heart.

For your cardiac muscle to be fit and healthy you'll want to eventually add calm, intelligent bouts of cardio two to three times a week, again, right at or under the 30-minute mark. As a culture we've been sold a bill of goods on cardio. It's not the most efficient caloric burn and it's not how you're going to change your physical body most effectively for the positive. In fact, it can often have the exact opposite effect, most particularly because of hormone balance.

Cardio for wellness and well-rounded fitness can be as simple as walking, hiking, interval training, Tabata, swimming, or my preferred method - jumping on a mini rebounder, also known as a trampoline.

Rebounding is the unsung hero of cardio. It's my favorite because it's so smart, efficient, and still underappreciated and unknown. Rebounding has so many benefits: It increases bone density. It's kind on your joints. Just 20 minutes of rebounding has the same benefits as a full hour of running. It's one of the most effective and efficient ways to detoxify the lymphatic system. It increases coordination and reaction times. It's endorsed by NASA. Yes, *that* NASA. NASA states it's the best cardio you can do and um, yeah, they're pretty smart so I'm with NASA on this one, plus it's fun!

Regardless of the physical benefits, if you suffer from seasonal depression, depression, or general cranky moods, high-stress jobs or lives it is a happiness maker. You simply can't be in a bad mood after jumping. I have my kids use it and it's a lifesaver in the winters in New York.

Rebounding also passively strengthens the pelvic floor and let's be frank, if you've had children, you need this and are too afraid to talk about it or ask what you can do to improve the leaking that occurs postnatal. If you have a tendency to leak … this strengthens those muscles, the pelvis floor, to allow strengthening and healing. The leaking can stop. The pelvic floor is simply a muscle that can and should be strengthened. Rebounding does it like no yoni egg, ben wa balls, or kegels can.

Not to mentions the benefits of heightened sensation during sex and stronger orgasms with a stronger pelvic floor. Yup. Jumping on a trampoline improves your sex life. Pilates also contributes to this, because of the attention to core contraction, getting #onthemat with me will strengthen your pelvic floor too.

If you embark on rebounding you'll want a rebounder with bungee cords not springs for the care and benefit of your joints.

If you love cardio and simply can't imagine life without it, it's your jam and your joy, I'm not here to rain on your parade. Joy is worth so much in your wellness and I'm clear that for every rule there is an exception and duality is real, but if you hate cardio, despise running — 1. Why are you doing it?! And 2. You don't need to and I'm going to tell you why. Let me start by saying — stop doing things you hate because you think you should — a life lesson that applies to all things. Loving something always reaps better rewards because of your focus and mindset. Unicorns are simply not about beating themselves up and they know the power of focus is downright magical. Where your focus goes energy flows so when you dislike something the energy is just negative around it no matter how good it's supposed to be for you.

Here are some truths about running and intense cardio, in particular for female bodies; running long distances — anything over 30 minutes non-stop — triggers a stress response in our bodies. After 30-minutes at a medium to high intensity of any cardio a body *thinks* what you are doing is about fight or flight — that you're being chased by a bear or are in danger of injury or death — cortisol gets produced and has a hay-day. Cortisol stashes in your belly and can either create a little pooch there or keep the weight that's already there firmly in place.

Cortisol prevents weight loss and can even cause weight gain. It's not a hormone you want to be actively producing for your best fitness and wellness. When we talk about decreasing stress in your life for better health we're actually talking about decreasing cortisol levels. Cardio as a tool for your best fitness is a completely false paradigm. It's incredibly hard on the skeletal system and becomes even more so with time — yes, as we age. It's also imperative for those of us with autoimmune systems, or suspected autoimmune issues, cling to this information about cardio. Blowing out our adrenals, producing cortisol or firing a fight or flight response in our system are the last things we need to be doing. It's actually harmful to us.

Remember, our physical bodies haven't evolved as far as our technologies have. Our bodies are still incredibly primal. The biological make up between male and female also adds to this conversation. Men, from a biological perspective are the hunter-gatherers. Women are multi-taskers who are designed to sprint but not for long distances.

One of the first steps with clients for nearly two decades now is to completely pull them off all cardio for three full months then calmly ween them back into it to allow for hormone balance. In particular to decrease cortisol and calm and bolster the adrenal glands and watch the magic of weight fall off simply because of hormonal balance.

You'll hear me continually repeat that body change happens in the rest stages … not in an actual workout. This is a classic example of how PR and marketing have confused the situation. Marketing wants you to run — runners spend money on shoes, shorts, trackers, registration fees for races, etc., etc. Walking requires far less and interval training doesn't wear and tear on a pair of shoes like distance running does and jumping on a trampoline is a one time purchase for the tramp and requires zero additional gear.

I suggest that on top of your four to six times a week #onthemat with me on matandkitchen.com, you layer in intelligent and kind cardio two to three times a week, no more than 30-minutes at a time of the above listed formats and if you go with the rebounder you'll only truly need two to 20 minutes for true results. Jumping is intense. You'll start small and build up to the full 20 minutes and if you have autoimmune issues you may stay in the two to 10 minute range depending on your adrenal levels.

Why Pilates?

I've worked in the fitness industry for nearly 20 years and practiced pilates for over 20 years. I'm an avid yogi and clearly have a yogic sensibility about my training, but I don't specifically teach yoga. My calling card and niche has always been in pilates, even when (especially when) it wasn't en vogue.

Pilates is the only fitness format that you can directly take to any other format. The same cannot be said for anything else. I've done them all, and even taught many of them for years. Pilates literally makes everything else you do better because of its roots in physical therapy, breath, alignment, form, and core connection. Any serious athlete or trainer will tell you that the strength of your core is truly worth its weight in gold when it comes to wellness and fitness. It prevents injury, heals existing injuries, allows you to train when injured, loosens what's tight and tightens what's loose, and gives you an athletic *edge* to every sport you play for fun or competition. Pilates creates a balanced body with "equal length and equal strength."

I teach mat workouts grounded in pilates because it's what bodies need the most. You will see other exercises and formats woven into my workouts but they are always grounded in the pilates method. In a nutshell, pilates is the most intelligent fitness format out there. And I'm all about efficient and smart. Life is meant to be lived, not wasted #onthemat. After All, unicorns have magic to do … they need to be efficient and balanced.

Isn't Yoga More 'Magical' Than Pilates?

Depends on who you're taking it from.

As in all things the intention and the source matters. Let's be honest, there's a skewed conversation when it comes to self-realization, magic, woo-woo, manifestation, and all things #highvibe. We've been sold this persona that you can only be magical if you're doing yoga. I'm here to contest that. In the hands of a gifted, intelligent, and deep yogi, yoga can be that. I've experienced it … but it can also be compressing, ill cued, not appropriate to the body it's working with (BIG TIME), and end up doing more harm than good because the instruction and messages you receive in the realm of yoga is all about a fab Instagram pic.

I've worked in the fitness industry for the greater part of my adult life and know that bodies that are rooted in pilates become beautiful yogis, inside and out. Pilates students have an intellect and awareness about their physicality that is typically only present in professional athletes. Pilates brews unicorn magic because of its intelligent and calm approach to all body types.

Magic lies in the practitioner and teacher, not the format. Unicorns are magical by their uniqueness … not because they follow the herd of mere horses. This topic could be another full handbook all its own and I'll only go so far as to say that by believing that yoga is the only way to balance energies, clear energetic blockages, root intentions in the physical realm, raise your vibration, clear your pineal gland, strengthen and deepen your intuition, connect to your guides, guardian angels, or higher self simply narrows your definition of possibilities, magic, divine connection, cosmic flow and manifestation. I would argue that the more aligned your bone and tissue structures are, the better all the energetic pathways flow and light up. When you focus on alignment and form and working with the way a body is built to thrive rather than forcing it into shapes it's not prepared to yet approach, you evolve your personal magic more effectively and efficiently.

And yes, the above is my point of view. Learning to work with your body rather than against it is exactly what brews unicorn magic.

Add in the topic of your solar plexus chakra and where it is — at your center. Your core. The *I am*, manifesting central portion of your physical body. Pilates, as a format addresses this above all else. Strengthening your core, coming from your center, moving with focused attention at your center AT ALL TIMES. To truly wrangle to stars and draw your manifestations into fruition you must be deeply and powerfully grounded at your root, sacral and solar plexus chakras. You can open and lift your third eye and crown chakras but if they are unanchored you won't get much more than visions, vivid dreams, anxiety, and potentially panic attacks from the ungrounded energies you're running.

Can we see how engaging mula bandha a few times in a yoga practice might pale in comparison to always initiating and beginning with a deep, stable, uplifted core contraction with every movement? Mic. drop.

Feeling Good is More Important Than Looking Good

The benefits of working out are about how you feel and what your system is capable of doing, not simply how you look. How you feel affects EVERYTHING in your life. Especially when you're a unicorn. Our feels are our internal moral compass. How we feel directly impacts our capacity to *know* and hear what our intuition is telling us. We need clean and clear systems so messages are running on clear and open lines of communication. If you're an empath, highly sensitive, or flat out psychic (and we all are … most of us just need to cultivate our psychic muscles — our intuition) you know this to be true. You need a lot of water to run these higher vibrations and energies. You require quiet, calm, and down time. You must move your body with intention because we are magical beings having a physical experience. You need high speed, unencumbered chi — like techies need high speed internet in order to run code at adept speeds — unicorns need open, primed and anchored bodies to receive messages, signs, symbols, and omens with clarity and confidence.

We're training to be unicorns because by improving ourselves, we improve the world. We shine brighter and happier and to do that we've got to initiate from our core, move from our center and find balance in both the physical and metaphysical. Unicorns must workout. Consistently. And most of the movement has nothing to do with the physical, but with the universal energies coming and going.

Unicorns have more patience, energy, focus, clarity of thought, creativity, and happier attitudes. The benefits of becoming a unicorn are about so much more than a calorie burned or what size pants you're wearing. What we accomplish #onthemat directly impacts what we accomplish #offthemat. How you feel on the inside is far more important than what the packaging looks like on the outside.

Unicorns transmute fitness into wellness. When you consistently practice wellness, fitness comes … the same is not true in reverse.

Meet Yourself on the Mat

No matter what fitness level you are entering your unicorn training with, approach each video with me with fresh eyes. Do what *YOUR* body is capable of that day, **Do as much of a video as you can!** Two minutes, five minutes, 15 or the full 30. It's about getting *BETTER*. It's about doing *BETTER* and creating wellness and feeling empowered.

Becoming a unicorn may happen in increments for you. **Meet yourself on the mat.** You'll hear me say this a lot in the workouts at www.unicornwellnessstudio.com. We all need reminders not to compare ourselves. We are each on our own, unique journey. As a teacher, I'm simply farther along the path than my students. I've been up ahead with a flashlight for years, laying mile markers and setting up snacks and water, moving branches off the trail so your path is easier.

Simply listen to my cues during your workout and allow those cues to translate in your body the best they can, each workout. It's *never* about doing what I can do, it's about giving it your best, showing up, seeing what you can do in that workout *today*, getting consistent in your practice and getting better in the long run. Working out with me is about cultivating awareness and connection. Working out with me is about having a conversation with your body. Not simply taking your body through the motions. Anyone can do that. Unicorns don't phone it in.

To truly be a unicorn you must be compassionate, connected, present, and in a working relationship with our physical body. We are spiritual beings having a physical experience and we must tend to the physical components with respect and consistency, all the while knowing we are so much more than this body. Always start calm and small and build to the big for long term success. Everyone is coming at this from a different place. Honor that.

ASSIGNMENT 2 : HYDRATION

If any one thing is going to turn you into a unicorn … IT'S WATER! If you learn nothing else from me, you should learn the importance of water for your body.

1. Drink 8 ounces of warm water (yes, the warm matters, it's easier for your body to process and flushes mucus more efficiently) with lemon juice every morning before you eat or drink anything else. Cut a lemon in half and squeeze it into your cup. Yes, it needs to be a real lemon. No essential oils. No concentrates. Real. Lemon.

2. Hydrate your body with half of your body weight in ounces of water a day. Not tea, coconut water, nor bubble or sparkling waters, just still, filtered, bought, tap, or boiled simple WATER. Alkaline is best, but don't let this be an excuse or a hurdle … work with whatcha got. If tap is what you have, go with that to begin with.

Note: #betterISbetter on this one. If you have a challenging time getting your full ounces of water each day, get as close to it as you can and work your way up to the full ounces, hopefully by the end of four weeks but longer if need be.

Water is Essential

Sixty to 70 percent of your body is made up of water. Eighty-five percent of your brain tissue is water. It's the only liquid we need in order to thrive and survive, everything else is simply want or entertainment. Don't get me wrong, I drink coffee, I drink an occasional alcoholic beverage but I know those are fun and celebratory and more about my emotions or my soul not feeling deprived than for my optimal health.

Water is Necessary

Hydration flushes your system of daily toxins. It keeps things running smoothly and prevents your system from getting sick. Flushing your system energizes you, allows you to workout stronger and even longer. Water is essential for healthy digestion and nutrient absorption, and it lubricates your joints to take away and prevent pain.

Unicorns run on water. Water is free. It's simple. It cuts down on caloric intake, it alleviates that afternoon energy slump when you typically grab another cup of coffee or high sugar treat to keep you going. You could lose 2 to 15 lbs. (depending on your body) simply by getting hydrated because you're flushing out all the detritus in your system. Literally.

A hydrated body is perkier and more focused. Water hydrates the brain tissue and makes you more alert and aware. Water plumps the skin and improves fine lines and acne. Water improves cardiovascular health by increasing blood volume. Water greatly influences your flexibility, mobility, and joint health. That crunchy sound in your knee? You might just need to get hydrated for it to be alleviated.

The list goes on and on and the simple magic of hydration is real.

Unicorns require copious amounts of water to sparkle and shine. And the woo-woo recommendation on hydration is even more powerful: highly sensitive, intuitive, psychic bodies require ample hydration to *run* the kinds of energy they are receiving and processing. Yes, I said this about movement as well … see how this whole Unicorn Handbook thing is playing out? Taking care of our physical bodies has a direct relation to our capacity to connect with the divine, our intuition, our higher selves, God. Call it what you will but how we tend to our physical body is in direct relation to our respect of our divine connection and this physical incarnation. We've been loaned this physical home, it's nothing but respectful of the divine to take care of it in the best of ways, to the best of our knowledge. Water is a biggie to us unicorns.

Why Lemon in the Water?

Lemon water has a whole other set of sparkling benefits to help you feel amazing and capable all day long. One of it's main benefits is that it boosts your metabolism if you drink it first thing in the morning. You'll actually burn more calories throughout your day. Lemon water alkalizes your body. Alkaline systems are healthier and create an environment that does not breed sickness (especially cancer). It's excellent for your colon, gallbladder, and liver functions and lowers general inflammation in the body. Lowering inflammation is HUGE for fitness results and overall health. — More on this in your Fuel section below.

WEEK TWO

In week two we gallop towards a food education that will change the way you look at nutrition, food, and fuel.

ASSIGNMENT 3 : FUEL

What we put in our mouths and bodies matters. Food has become such an emotional issue that we often forget about its actual function. Food's true function is fuel. Bodies are designed to thrive on food from the earth. We cultivate glowing health from the nutrients, vitamins, and minerals that our bodies extract from food, food that is as "un-messed with" (unprocessed) as possible. Nothing more and nothing less. When the balance of real food is off, our bodies speak to us in excess weight, inflammation, headaches, terrible sleep, chronic issues, disorders, disease, depression, and anxiety.

How to Feed a Unicorn

Unicorns represent the convergence of the brute strength of a workhorse with the lightness of purity and magic. Fueling a unicorn is simple: Aim for pure ingredients, whole real foods that bolster, nourish, and support. Stay far away from packaged and processed products masquerading as food.

Read my 41 Day Food Reset at the back of this handbook. Consider doing it. If you've read it before, read it again. If you've done it before, consider doing it again. You will learn something new about yourself every single time you read it or do it. Everyone learns something from the process — typically, something unexpected and highly valuable. And no, I'm not being dramatic or exaggerating. It's a food adventure that any true unicorn needs to embark on at least once in their lives.

Pick one smoothie in the Unicorn Wellness 'Kitchen' (after logging into your account at www.unicornwellnessstudio.com) or from the Reset. Could you pick a smoothie from somewhere else? Sure, just make sure it's as pure and clean as you can get, no boxed alternative milks, no guar gum, carrageenan, inulin, or peanut butter. Clean is the overall name of the fueling game. No dairy, no protein powders, and preferably organic ingredients. Have this smoothie every morning this week after your warm lemon water OR prepare one or two eggs (pasture raised is best) with a breakfast salad. You'll see these on my

Instagram @tandy_gutierrez often. Any handful of greens will do plus any veggies you'd like to add. My typical breakfast is arugula or kale with sauteed broccoli, cherry tomatoes, yellow bell peppers, beets, and half of an avocado with pink salt. Pick what speaks to you and what your lifestyle allows for.

Simplify - If you don't embark on the ultimate unicorn adventure of my Food Reset right away, choose one or more of the tactics below to layer into these four weeks.

Go GREEN! Greens are the easiest internal coolers and cleansers. Add a handful to every meal this week. Doesn't matter what kind and yes, this includes breakfast or smoothies. I tell my kids that greens are the internal scrubbers of the body. Greens truly keep us sickness- and disease-free. They increase your energy in major ways and they also have a huge impact decalcifying your pineal gland … yup, to improve your third eye, intuition, personal unicorn horn growth. Unicorns thrive on greens.

Up Your Veggies. No, not your fruits. If you're a major fruit eater try swapping a portion or three of your fruits for a veggie this week. Fruits are sugars, even if they are real and they are not meant to be our major source of energy or nutrients. Bodies thrive on veggies. It's how our physical system is designed. And no, I'm not a vegan or a vegetarian. Zero judgment for those of you who are, it's just simply not how my personal system thrives best. Our physical bodies are built to thrive on veggies. Veggies stabilize blood sugar and balance hormones. They energetically root and ground us. They keep us thriving and even-keeled. Too much sugar, even if it's real, can still have us riding an insulin roller-coaster and potentially whisk us off to the ethers making it hard to focus or receive clear messaging. In order to become a unicorn with a high vibe and strong, clear intuition, you've actually got to get more grounded (also another vote for consistently working out). You must be rooted in your physical body in order to fully connect with the divine. Getting too zippy and ungrounded you simply cannot be of full service to the greatest good of all involved. This is why I have to keep animal protein in my personal diet — when I don't, I zip off into the ethers, like a little unicorn-shaped balloon unable to focus, riddled with anxiety and insomnia. This isn't the case with everyone, but again, it's a vote for cracking your own food code via the Reset to discover what makes your personal unicorn tick rather than trying to feed your unicorn either what mere horses eat, or another unicorn's fuel. We're each unique and need to discover for ourselves what best supports our personal strain of magic.

Cook and or pack more of your meals this week than you typically do. This one is simple. If you never cook or pack a lunch, try it once. There is so much that happens by physically connecting with your food. I am an energetic person. I am an empath. I firmly believe that energy is passed in everything we do and that cooking with love, handling your own food, understanding the process and getting anchored to it matters. Things that are processed by machines, sealed in plastic, and shuttled quickly along metal conveyor belts are packed with additives and junk and, yes, carry an icky-drag-you-down-low energy. Unicorns simply don't exist on these types of foods. Cooking and packing your own food gives you connection, pride, and empowerment with what's in it. Even the healthiest of packaged options are often loaded with sneaky bits that are undermining your best efforts at harnessing your inner unicorn.

Leave off a sauce. Simple. Skip the ketchup. Nix the mayo and dump the dressing. Unless you made your own, or read the label in depth, these things are land mines of additives and the major monsters: refined sugar, gluten, HFCS, and corn. Do this for as many meals as you are willing to try. Or swap out your need to cover or drown your food for simple additions like olive oil, coconut oil, flax oil, vinegar, lemon, lime, blood orange, herbs, and pink salt or fresh pepper. Skip the sea salt. If you haven't heard the news yet …

it's proving to be packed with micro bits of plastic because our poor oceans are filled with the stuff. Unicorns simply can't stomach plastic.

The reality of food is that as a culture we make it complicated. It's not. Eating whole real foods will generate a body that is healthy #fromtheinsideout. Eating whole real foods will generate a unicorn.

To Make a Major Impact on Your Eating, Embrace Simplicity

Allow food to be simple. Less saucy, less layers. Just less. Think assembly rather than cooking. Your outsides reflect, directly, what you are fueling with on the inside. Though this may not always be easy, it is simple.

Even for those eating healthy, if your outsides don't reflect your inner unicorn, either you're not eating as well as you think, you're not being honest with yourself about what you're eating you're eating real, whole foods that are simply not in accordance with your personal food code. This is addressed in full in the Reset at the end of this handbook: Just 'cause something is healthy doesn't mean it's a fit for you, or your hormones need some major assistance in balancing — again, a vote for getting #onthemat with me and pressing play and doing the Reset.

If you do not sparkle and shine, something isn't a fit. There is an imbalance in the system somewhere. And if all the physical possibilities are being addressed and your best unicorn self still isn't shining through, then we address your energy, your spirit, your emotions, and we work from the inside out on the energetic level to heal, peel, and repair layers to cultivate your best self in meditation and through the self-evolution available through the tarot.

Perk up your choices in these four weeks if the full Reset isn't in the stars right now. Assist your body's natural processes of elimination and build on the wins. Add a few of the options above to your week;

don't get stressed or complicate things. Unicorns focus on the long term and take calm steps in that direction without spooking themselves.

A General Unicorn Feeding Note

I'm a huge fan of smoothies or eggs and greens in the morning, salads with protein at lunch, and cooked proteins and veggies with greens at night.

Play, enjoy, think of your food as an experiment in simplicity. How many veggies can you infuse your plate with? How many colors can you fill your meals with? What can you leave off because you're wanting it for entertainment or emotional comfort rather than hunger or nutritional fuel?

I encourage you to shift your perspective around "healthy" eating (this term makes me crazy — it's just eating the way our bodies are designed to) from deprivation, diet, or punishment to releasing what doesn't work for your system. You'll make space in your life for other thoughts and pursuits … 'cause if you're not micromanaging calories or deciding what foodie thing to experience and post about next you've got waaaay more time to focus on a literal world out there.

Decluttering your food closet creates space for new ideas and fresh endeavors. Paring down the elements of your plate allows you to focus and create for the greater good of the world. It gives you more time and clarity to think, make, and do.

By only fueling with what makes your engine hum, your outsides sparkle and shine and your immune system becomes hearty and bolstered while your body finds its personal best set point with weight.

The whole, real foods thing is going to be a broken record, get used to it. Unicorns don't do fake, fillers, synthetic, cheap, or low vibe.

Real is Always Best

Ditch the fast food, prepared meals, boxed and packaged products and start adding more real, whole foods to your days. You can never go wrong with the real deal. Unicorns don't eat junk.

Eat breakfast, lunch, and dinner. Eating three meals a day will keep insulin levels stable, your metabolism stoked, and moods cheery. Try not to wait longer than four hours to eat to avoid dropping your insulin levels and, crashing your energy, mood, and metabolism.

And no, I can't come and cook it for you. Part of the point of the Reset is to reconnect on a physical, tangible level with your food. There's a lot to be said for cooking with love and handling and preparing your own meals. It's a method of grounding in and of itself. Touching and prepping the elements of the earth is important, necessary, and powerful.

I didn't grow up cooking. In fact, I only really started six years ago. See, there's hope for you too! It was only by embracing my wellness journey that I cultivated the skill of cooking. I teach it because if I can learn — just ask my husband about my kitchen skills prior to writing the Reset (I literally burned everything) — then anyone can. We can all do the things we wish we could. Unicorns acknowledge our wishes as wants and predestined accomplishments and then get down to practicing fearlessness (doing things in spite of fear) and embracing the adventure of learning and always stepping up to meet the universe halfway to our wishes. Unicorns keep their eyes on the prize more than on the burden of doing the work to reach the prize.

Learn to Listen to Your Body

Remember, becoming a unicorn is about self-awareness, intuition, self-respect, and self-trust. How you fuel is a conversation with your body, not an argument. Becoming a unicorn is about the union of intellect with intuition. This is the BIGGEST piece of your magical transformation. Learning that your personal messaging and wiring eclipses all other messaging. Transitioning to more real food is deeply anchored in a conversation with our bodies. It's a transition from being at war with ourselves to being on a journey with it.

Food has become super emotional in our modern culture, but it doesn't have to be. It wasn't always. It used to be simply about fueling, sustaining life. Food was once about what we had. What we grew, what was near, or what could be traded for.

If you are at the beginning of your food journey, it may feel complicated and it can Get. Very. Emotional. If you allow yourself the opportunity for a food adventure via the Reset, you can transition out of these emotional bonds with foods that no longer serve you — that have never served you. These emotional bonds with foods are in complete opposition to your best self. Your best self knows it simply needs nourishment and bolstering. The modern emotional bonds with food do not allow you to be a unicorn. Emotional bondage by food puts a big ole corral around your unicorn spirit. It's time to ditch the emotional tethers. Unicorns are bound by nothing. They roam free through the light of the cosmos.

In order to fully become a unicorn you need to be willing to release all you've learned about food, all you think you know about nutrition and diets you've done in the past. In order to truly become a unicorn you'll need a firm footing in potential, change, metamorphosis, mutation, and a true belief that the best sparkling and shining self is possible for everyone. Including you. You'll need to be open to what works for you now — in this body, at this time, in this moment. Not what worked for you years ago or what works for your sister, best friend or co-workers. Unicorns are utterly unique, each and every one of us.

Unicorns embrace and love that they are like no one and nothing else. Allow yourself to discover what you need now, in this moment at this time, free of expectations and free of the past stories or experiences. Allow yourself to be you, at this moment in time, perhaps for the first time in this lifetime.

The Reset

While whole real foods are always the answer to a fit and healthy body, the exact details can be very different from person to person. Each person is a spectacular, individual expression of themselves. Everyone is their own majestic unicorn. We are each made up of different genetic, experiential, medical, emotional, numerical, and energetic layers. No two of us are alike, so neither is the food we need in order to balance and thrive within our gorgeous, unique body.

I created the 41 Day Food Reset to heal myself. I never intended to share it. Friends, members, clients, and followers saw how my health was transitioning and asked if they could do it as well. I hesitated in a major way because I'm not a doctor, nutritionist, or dietitian. I don't have a bunch of extra letters behind my name so I figured I wasn't worthy and no one would take me as an *expert* on this topic. Yup, I have very non-unicorn moments. But as I shared it with one person at a time, I saw the results, the epiphanies, the healing, weight loss, and the unbelievable discoveries that people had been hunting for, just as I had been. After incredible feedback and health transformations, we added it to the membership offering, online. I continue to be grateful to be a part of others healing and empowerment process. I'm forever grateful for this protocol to have come through me to help others.

Think of me as your earth momma, kitchen witch, highly read and researched wellness nerd BFF that wants to share anything and everything that could make healing and positive body evolution more efficient and accessible for you.

The Reset delves deep. Evolving to your best self can be uncomfortable (think cocoon and butterfly). Becoming your best self, a unicorn, will challenge some of your thoughts about family, friends, and those who *love* you. It will poke at how and if they support you as you explore other ways of doing things, especially around food. Your connections to food are about so much more than just *you*. If you do embark on cracking your own food code, you'll start to look at the whole picture not just the plate in front of you.

Take one step at a time. You're standing at the bottom of the staircase and your goals are at the top. Doing the Reset is merely a step on the route up. Don't skip stairs, you can't navigate around one floor or another. Simply place one foot at a time, one in front of the other as you climb your Reset staircase. Your goals are at the top. Completely within reach but you have to do the doing, you'll need to do the Reset at some point in order to get there.

You have to learn new things and new ways of being in order to be new. It will take practice and faith. You may not always enjoy each step of the process, but you will love standing at the top of that staircase. There is nothing comparable to the feeling of being your best self, honoring your system.

There is nothing better than being a unicorn.

Food has the power to heal #fromtheinsideout. I'm living proof. The power of food is underrated and often overlooked as "too much work." I'll tell you what's too much work: sickness, endless doctors appointments, paying for those appointments, chemical medications, dealing with insurance companies and even, in extreme cases, surgeries.

Food has the power to prevent and heal if we simply give it a chance to do what is was designed to do in harmony with our body.

Wellness Through Food Awareness

Bloating, gas, acne, headaches, and stomach cramps are not *normal*. They are signals that certain foods are not a fit for your body. They are signals from your body that it needs balance, bolstering, support, and nurturing. They are also seriously un-unicorn-like. These are signs that something is off. It's a mode of communication from your body to you.

When you crack your own food code and buy what works for your body, you allow yourself to fully transform into a unicorn. You allow the best version of yourself to show up in the world strong, healthy, vibrant, and full of joy.

If you take out the things that don't work, regardless of how *healthy* they are or what tribe you believe yourself to belong to (omnivore, paleo, vegan, vegetarian, etc.)

you will start to feel more like a unicorn and in turn begin to look more like one … because what we *wear* on our insides is what we *wear* on our outsides. This goes for emotions, beliefs, rest, self-care, and the ultimate … fuel.

You simply have to be willing to discover what those foods are and practice abiding by them. You must have faith that things will work for the best outcome. You must know that our bodies are built to thrive, we've simply been treating them poorly for too long. We've been feeding ourselves like we're mere horses, rather than magical unicorns.

It's time to fuel like a unicorn with simple, whole, real foods that are overflowing with nourishing, tantalizing, satiating, and supportive components.

WEEK THREE

In week three we slow down to allow for true transformation through self-care education that will change the way you think about rest, myofascial release, and bathing.

ASSIGNMENT 4: SLEEP

Unicorns know that they have big days ahead of them. They also never know when they will be needed most, that they must be ready at a moment's notice to protect and heal. They tend to their systems for the long game in order to always be ready when needed. Think of your inner unicorn as the best friend or momma that is always supportive and present. Fundamental preparation of a unicorn begins with a restored and rested system. Sleep deprivation has a proven adverse impact on overall reaction times, capacity to think clearly, and capacity for internal systems to act

properly. Don't let a sleep imbalance catch you off guard preventing your mythical self from emerging. Learn to sleep better in order to become a unicorn.

Sleep is Essential

When we sleep our bodies cleanse, restore, and regenerate. Hormones are released, tissues repair and grow. We regulate our appetite hormones as well as consolidate memories for cognition. Bottom line: It's our reboot time and this is actually where positive change happens for our fitness and wellness. Working out, hydration, and eating well are great, but you won't reap the rewards unless you're rested.

Change of any kind, but most particularly physical change, does not occur in the moment, it occurs in your rest cycles. Meaning, you can eat well, workout, and hydrate but if you aren't sleeping well, your body won't change to the degree it can.

These transitions of fat loss, lean muscle growth, or even lowering your blood pressure ALL HAPPEN WHEN YOU REST. Everything else is preparation for change, not actual change.

Sleep affects everything — everything we do, our skin, our capacity to focus and think clearly, our physical reaction times, the strength of our immune system. All of it. If we're not sleeping well, we're not thriving. Our entire hormonal and digestive systems get a *clean sweep* and reset every evening. When we cut that process short, we're doing a huge disservice and disrespect to our systems #fromtheinsideout. When we're not tending to our sleep we are actually thwarting our own progress at becoming our most magical self.

It's also where we dream, where our subconscious is at its most receptive, and where we can catch full or fragmented messages from our intuition, guides, guardian angels, higher self, ancestors, and pure divine spirit.

Unicorns need their dream time for physical restoration and transformation, but they also need their dream time to connect to divine spirit. Sleep is practical magic. If you're not sleeping *enough* or well your poor body is not only suffering but your spiritual relationship is seriously missing out. Remember unicorns are deeply rooted in the real world but equally connected in the ethers. Sleep is where those two worlds are bridged.

How Much Sleep Should a Unicorn Get?

You need seven to nine hours of sleep a night. That being said, all systems are different and you'll need to do some trial and error to figure out where your *sweet spot* is. That sweet spot is defined as waking up feeling refreshed; it's that simple. It doesn't mean you're cheery or necessarily jumping out of bed. Some of us are quiet and slow to wake up (I am not in any way considered a morning person, I'm a Taurus sun and I will never bound radiantly from bed in the early a.m., but you should definitely feel rested.

You may not be able to achieve this every day, but we're looking for the law of averages when it comes to wellness. For example, my body loves and thrives with nine hours of sleep, sometimes as much as 10. That's not always realistic for my schedule, but I do try for that and know that when I'm in sleep deficit for the week I'm bound to not feel well. Those of us with chronic issues, diseases, or sensitive systems must take extra care to respect and protect our sleep.

Sleep is All About Transitions

We can't always get more sleep, but we can improve how quickly we get to sleep and improve the quality of our sleep once we're there. The goal is to get more deep sleep that's restorative and refreshing. Even if you're not a parent, you can understand the lengths one goes to in order to transition our kiddos to sleep. We introduce special blankets, lovies, bedtime stories, soft music, baths, and lavender laced lotions. Why in the world would we think that we are any different?

Learning to sleep is all about self-care and transitioning from the working world to solace. We need bedtime rituals, just like we set for our precious littles. We are no different. Our nervous systems need signals that say: calm down … quiet down … it's time to power down. Our modern tech-filled lives put up many hurdles in that transition. They're not insurmountable, but they require attention. Our response to cycles of light and dark (circadian rhythms) are natural. We are meant to wake when it's light out and sleep when it's dark. These circadian rhythms get severely hijacked by screens or overnight shifts, working odd hours, having infants who are still learning their circadian rhythms, etc. Much of what we do these days works against the capacity to sleep.

ASSIGNMENT 5 : BEDTIME RITUALS

Choose one or more of the bedtime rituals below. How many is up to you. Choose what speaks to you, what seems fun, calming, and grounding. Choose things that you will look forward to trying. Choose what sounds simple to implement. Do not choose what you think you *should* do or what everyone else has told you to do. Have fun, listen to your instincts.

Note: #betterisbetter If your bedtime rituals get too complicated, it won't work. The goal is to calm and relax your physical and nervous system and allow your body to rest, NOT to stress it out more and set the bar too high. Unicorns know their limitations. They are always up for a challenge but they acknowledge limitations. They aren't pegasus', they can't fly … they navigate just fine on the ground.

Unicorns have a horn growing from the center of their head. They absolutely own their uniqueness. Who cares if the rituals that work for you are silly or odd? Do they work? Then go with it. Branch out, try something new. Get outside your comfort zone and ENJOY the process.

1. **Set a "Cut Off" or Straight Up Bedtime** - Think about how many hours you think you need to be restored, count backwards from your wake-up time then do the best you can to abide by that to actually close your eyes to sleep. Yup. Unicorns set a straight up bedtime. Embracing your inner child is a key component of invoking your inner unicorn.

2. **Low Lights** - Approximately 30 minutes before bedtime, transition your world to low light, signaling it's time to wind down and rest. Candles work well. Amber, rose, or red light are the best to counterbalance the blue light of computer, phone

screens, and high-efficiency bulbs. Fun ways to introduce amber and rose light into your life include pink salt lamps, just turn it on in the evening, at least 30 minutes before bed in the room you'll be in, you can turn the dimmer down and sleep with it on as well. Amber colored glasses might not look or feel super cool but you can continue to read or work on a screen or watch while still winding down. You can do a simple online search to find amber glasses, plus there are loads of settings on your devices that will swap the lights on your screens to a *nighttime* version for you.

3. **Warm Water** - It's a plain old comforting. Thirty to 60 minutes before your bedtime take a bath with one to two cups of Epsom salts for muscle relaxation and hydration. Stay in 15 to 40 minutes for the full benefit. If baths aren't your thing, a shower or a simple cup of caffeine-free tea will do. Transition your system with

warm, comforting things that signal your system to slow down. More info on the benefits and magic of Epsom baths in Assignment 5.

4. **Sound** - Try listening to a guided meditation or binaural beats with a set of headphones. This is a favorite way of mine to fall asleep or when flying for travel. It's a passive way to meditate and a wonderful way to take care of your brain and body. Pick one that works for you — there unlimited choices out there, just do a little searching online. Unicorns are highly meditated and binaural beats are the easiest entry point, in my opinion. Binaural beats are "auditory illusions" … seeeeeeee magic already. … They are frequencies you listen to in headphones, one frequency is played in one ear, while another is played in the other and your brain hears the *third* frequency that the combination creates. Just like meditation, binaural beats increase gray matter in your brain, they do what's called "hemi-

syncing" and allowing the left and the right side of the brain to *talk* to each other more easily. They are excellent for those with ADHD, anxiety, and depression. They increase your vibration in the true unicorn fashion and create more focus, calm, rest, and yes *intellect*. Hemi-synced brains are more efficient. If there is only one unicorn rest wagon you hop on … this one is it.

5. **Scent** - Essential oils are a powerful tool. I encourage you to explore essential oils for a ton of reasons if you haven't already, but sleep might be the most compelling reason to embark on them. Buy organic when you can. You want the highest quality oils you can get. Unicorns are built out of purity, as they represent true, infinite purity. Their fuel and the products that they slather themselves in reflect that. Unicorns keep things simple and pure with anything and everything. Embracing essential oils to help invoke your inner unicorn can

look like many things; dab a drop or two on your pillow before bedtime, diffuse in the room via a diffuser 30 to 60 minutes prior to bed or even make a room spray of 8 oz. of distilled water plus eight to 10 drops of your preferred scent. Lavender is the most common calming, sleep inducer but feel free to use any oil that is soothing to you. My personal recommendations for becoming a unicorn are: frankincense, rose, vanilla, lavender, and ylang-ylang but, as always, we are all utterly unique unicorns so pick what works for you. Get all of your senses involved in calming down. You can also toss a few drops of essential oils in your bath or on the floor of your shower. I tend to simply slather them on my palms, feet, forearms, and chest. More on essential oils later in the handbook.

6. **Weighted Blankets** - These are more unknown but getting a lot of attention lately. There is great

research coming out about blankets weighing 5 to 25 lbs. for making major improvements for insomnia and anxiety. I have not personally used one, but I want one! My family and I traveled for 10 months with one suitcase and one backpack each … we are committed to keeping our belongings minimal but of the highest quality, so they last. There wasn't room for a full size version but I do use a mini version of one and have for years, when I travel, I fly with one on my lap. The version I use can be heated up or just used for the weight. My kids love them too. Think of them as oversized eye pillows. They're like a warm unicorn nuzzle or a faux hug. They are calming simply because of their weight … and the fact that they mimic much of the effect of a hug.

Clearly there are other choices as well that you could create in the realm of ritual. You are not limited to my suggestions. They are meant to inspire. Feel free to be creative, spend time journaling, in prayer, stretching,

with watercolors, doing a
www.unicornwellnessstudio.com stretch
video, reading a book rather than a tablet,
or listening to music. What calms you
down? What relaxes you? How do you
want to end your day and seal it up and
send it on its way? Meditation before
bedtime is always an excellent choice as
well … we'll talk about that in Assignment
6.

If you wake up in the middle of the night
also try using one of your chosen tools to
get back to sleep.

Unicorn days are full of giving, doing, and
working. It's only fair and fitting that we
take a moment to say thank you or even
good riddance to it and restore ourselves
for what lies ahead in the next waking
hours. Sleep is about being calm and
allowing yourself to be vulnerable. Sleep is
the ultimate self-care and self respect. Like
all things, it takes a bit of effort and practice
to teach yourself how to do it and allow
your system to get the hang of it but it's
well worth it. Unicorns know when to nestle

into the woods and restore before bounding off to be magical and fearless again.

Unicorns aren't immortal

What?! I thought that was the whole gig, you say … after all they are magical and majestic. Nope, sorry. They're grounded in earthly pitfalls. They may be majestic, mythical beasts but they can be taken down when their most unique feature, their horn, is removed — or by anything poisonous or that restricts oxygen (just like us). Though magical, unicorns have weaknesses. They must protect and care for themselves in all the usual ways and perhaps even have to take more care of themselves. Sadly, anything magical will be sought and potentially hunted for sport. Not

to get too grim but as magical as we all
are, we still live in an earthy, human plane.

Unicorns take excellent care of themselves
finding beautiful places to rest, wash, and
feed in natural environments. They balance
their keen intellect and divine intuition to
navigate how and when they present
themselves. And they hide or retreat when
they need to restore — or to avoid those
with less-than-divine intentions and
energies. Unicorns never back down or
give up, even if they take a timeout, they
protect, replenish, thrive, and survive.
Unicorns are the ultimate symbol of the
combination of intellect, grounded reality,
and divine intuition.

The assignments in this handbook are the
convergence of intellect and intuition.
These habits are the magic you invoke
when you need more bolstering and
support in day-to-day life. Unicorns know

their strengths but are keenly and equally aware of their weaknesses. Those weaknesses are what will cause them to fail themselves and the hope they represent.

As Audre Lourde — writer, poet, feminist, and civil rights activist — so eloquently put it "Caring for myself is not self-indulgence, it is self-preservation, and that is an act of political warfare."

Self-care is not self-indulgence

Self-care is mandatory for unicorns, and the more you do it in life — and depending on what your body is comprised of (chronic issues, totally healthy, toxic relationships, less than ideal work situations, complicated family dynamics, etc.) you may need more self care in order to reach or maintain a balanced and healthy body. Remember that a body does not produce change or results unless it has ample rest. Change in a body; weight loss, hormone balance, strength increase, flexibility increase, health upswing, out right healing, career goals, life goals, adventures — in other words manifesting — can only happen at *rest*. You require self-care in order to reap the benefits of your work. Unicorns must take care in order to meet the universe halfway to their wishes.

ASSIGNMENT 6: SELF-CARE

Choose one of the self-care components below and up the amount it shows up in your life this week. i.e. one to six times … whatever works in your world. Meaning, if you've never done any of these, do it at least once. If you already have these in your routine, try having a full week of self-care. Explore.

Epsom Salt Detox Bath

Epsom salt baths are an extreme multitasker for a body. They ease stress, relax muscles, and calm the nervous system, detox the body of all things low vibe and muck making, and relieve pain and muscle cramps. If you soak for 15 minutes you get these benefits, but if you stay for a full 40 minutes you have pulled toxins out of the body and allowed your system to reabsorb the magnesium to hydrate your body and balance your insulin levels, as well as prevent hardening of arteries and increase blood and therefore oxygen levels in your body. This is always my first line of body defense for weekly maintenance or at any hint of sickness for my entire family.

Why do you think unicorns are always depicted coming in or out of an ocean? The Last Unicorn, anyone??

Epsom salt baths also play a huge role in cleansing your aura and stripping wayward energies that may have attached to us and are draining energy or mental clarity. If you already know you have spiritual gifts — and we ALL do, it just depends to what degree, how well they are tended to, utilized, and naturally show up in a person — such as clairvoyance, clairsentience, claircognizance … any of the clairs…. psychic knowing, highly sensitive or majorly empathetic … you NEED at least one weekly Epsom salt bath in your life to take the energetic strain off of your energetic body. It's an incredible tool for those of us with autoimmune issues as well. Why? Well, that's another book — I see those of us with highly sensitive bodies as those with highly gifted psychic talents that haven't been nurtured or balanced.

Yes, you can do a foot soak in place of a full bath if you live in a drought area, or would like to conserve water or don't have a bath or simply concerned at the water usage. You'll get the benefits but not the maximum benefit of muscle recovery.

And YES! If you live near the ocean, simply GO GET IN!

*Note: Add 1-2 cups of Epsom salts to a warm bath and soak 15 minutes for the muscle recovery benefit and 40 minutes for hydration. Bonus points for using Himalayan pink salt or adding one to six drops of essential oil to the water.

Stretching

Stretch when you don't feel like working out, when your mood is less than majestic or you feel sluggish or are recovering from a sickness.

Too many people skip stretching in their wellness life. Mostly because they're "not good at it" … um, hello … that's exactly the reason to do it! Your body needs this as a balance piece, intensely, if you are not flexible. I post two full 30-minute stretch videos near the new moon every month on www.unicornwellnessstudio.com to make sure you're getting it in the cycle of your training.

Stretching is more magical than you know. Here's why: You get so many of the same benefits as a full strength workout but it's even more kind on the body, decreased risk of injury, reduced low back pain, improved posture, increased circulation, increased blood flow, increased coordination, improved range of motion, increased energy, and improved coordination. And I'm just going to go ahead and say it, as we mature — Age — as we age, we lose elasticity in our skin, muscles, ligaments and tendons and a truly healthy body is balanced in strength and mobility. When you stretch and do workouts #onthemat with me you increase and maintain the suppleness of your system from the inside out. My workouts address your bones, muscles, ligaments, tendons, and fascia. As the saying goes *those who bend never break.* It becomes increasingly important to our wellness that we create or maintain mobility. Stretching does that for you. Working out with www.unicornwellnessstudio.com does that for you.

Myofascial Release a.k.a. Self massage and in our case Foam Rolling

Self Massage unlocks a unicorns truest magical attributes.

Foam rolling is basically the "poor man's massage." It's not a replacement for skin-to-skin contact of a gifted massage therapist but it can keep your visits fewer and farther between or really help the healing or strengthening process if massage isn't in your budget. Benefits include: improved lymph drainage, reduced muscle soreness, decreased risk of injury, improved posture, increased circulation, increased blood flow, improved coordination, and improved range of motion. This is another tool that is exponentially supportive to a system with autoimmune issues because of the benefits of lymph drainage and fascia recovery.

You can facilitate myofascial release with foam rollers or tennis balls. There is a world of products out there but simply always works.

To find your own foam rolling videos to work with search your UnicorWellness.Studio account:

1. Log in.
2. Click on 'My Account'
3. Enter keywords such as 'foam roller' 'myofascial' 'self massage' and it will pull all the videos in your personal account that include self massage.

If you don't have a foam roller workout yet, I rotate through all the props in perpetuity in the workouts … you'll get one soon! Just hang in there till it pops into the flow of videos. Or simply head over to my YouTube Channel to search for 'Tandy Gutierrez' and search for 'foam rolling' I have a couple there as well!

Contrast Shower

Running a little *hot-and-cold* periodically is a good thing.

A contrast shower is exactly what it sounds like. In the shower you'll alternate cold water with water that's as hot as you can manage. The *perfect* contrast shower would be one minute intervals of freezing cold water then one minute of hot-as-you-can-stand water. However, I teach #betterisbetter. For some (okay, for most) standing in freezing cold water for a minute sounds like a terrible punishment, even for a unicorn … start with what you can manage. Start your contrast showers with 10 seconds of each and add time as you practice this technique working your way up to a minute of each at a time for three to six cycles.

Why in the World Would you do This to Invoke your Inner Unicorn?

It's a scientifically solid method used as a training recovery technique for professional athletes. It's a stress management tool for a body. It's a wonderfully accessible multi-tasker that increases energy, detoxes the body (especially of lactic acid), and increases oxygen flow. The hot and cold water dilate and constrict blood vessels causing a wonderful pump of blood throughout the body. It also trains your body to withstand, tolerate, and recover from stress more quickly. It's great on a physical level as well as an energetic level. Stress comes in a wide range; physical, mental, or emotional. A contrast shower helps you recover faster, increases your energy, and adds a perk to your step. And if you're particularly *astral* and highly influenced by astrology and the planetary shifts (like I am) it's a wonderful tool to help manage access heat if your there's a particularly intense sun transit or, say, a grand fire trine lighting things up.

WEEK FOUR

In week four we go deeper and invite full evolution through spiritual ritual.

Unicorns are best known for the horn coming out of their forehead. The horn is what makes a unicorn a unicorn. This magical, mythical spiral is capable of bestowing incredible healing and historically was seen as the most valuable thing a king could possess. A unicorn horn is said to be the physical manifestation of intuition, your conscious or the higher self. It's a connection to the divine — creativity, flow, love, and yes, psychic *knowing*. Unicorn magic comes from the third eye, your sixth chakra, the pineal gland. A unicorn's horn is a strong, direct connection to the messaging of divine spirit … and you can cultivate your own.

I hear you, you're wondering if I've gone off the deep end with the unicorn metaphor. Hang in there. You came this far with me …

I'm a huge fan of bringing back ritual.

There is a profound benefit to physically *doing* things in repetition. We are after all, spiritual beings having a physical experience. We have bodies that require movement in order to be healthy, we must eat and drink in order to survive, and whether we like it or not we need to connect to something bigger, quieter, and more magical than ourselves.

It's important in our modern, tech-filled lives that we take time to be bored and to be quiet. We also need to proprioceptively connect to things (feel, touch, and process information from touching things with our hands and feet, in particular — another major reason I teach on the mat barefoot because it has greater impact to your overall health). Technology is wonderful, it's the blessing and the thing that has allowed me to connect with so many over the years, but it's only positive and useful in balance with our analog roots and tribal origins.

In our modern lives we don't connect through touch as much as in decades prior. As a culture we don't prepare our own food as often, we tap screens to pay for goods rather than exchanging money, palm-to-palm.

Spiritual ritual helps bridge the gap between the everyday tasks of living and doing in this earthly plane with the unlimited divine energies of the universe. Spiritual ritual gives you an opportunity to bring calm to your sympathetic nervous system, awareness to your thoughts and cultivate an open and receiving hotline for messages from your guides, guardians, angels, higher self, and straight up divine spirit. Spiritual ritual allows for contemplation and connection with the unseen energies we share our lives with and gives us the tools and eventually mastery to understand, navigate, and learn our lessons in this physical experience to be of the highest and greatest good with the least amount of damage. And though spiritual ritual sounds airy fairy it is the exact thing that allows us to root into what is truly real.

Spiritual ritual grounds and anchors us to the magic of existence.

Anything that sets a consistent practice of quiet in your life is valid as a spiritual ritual. Anything that allows for daydreaming, pondering, self-evaluation, self-reflection, digging into your place in the collective and the presence of the unknown is a spiritual ritual.

There are many ways of the unicorn, I'm sharing what has worked for me in unbelievably supportive, consistent, and nurturing ways. You can call the quiet, the knowing, the answers that arrive, anything you want. I call it magic.

Magic is the untouchable thing. It's hope, prayer, well wishes, good vibes, and … it's love. You simply can't be a unicorn without a connection to your personal fist full of glitter. Feeling that something good can happen any day at any moment is what gets us through the hard times and what creates the best times. Just like all good cartoons and fairy tales teach, if you can believe in magic you can achieve anything.

I'll tell you right now, I can train bodies all day long with exercises and eating the foods that abide by their personal food code but if their head and heart are not in a hopeful, slightly magical space that allows for change, believes in positive outcomes, and fully anticipates miracles … their body will never change. As a trainer in the fitness industry for two decades I can confidently state that where your head and heart reside is where true results occur. I've seen it in thousands of clients and in myself.

I offer up this section on spiritual ritual to get us connected and aware of not just ourselves, but to each other and to the unseen magic that exists in the world. I offer up this section because your wellness is not just about the physical body. It's about the collective unconscious agreements and energies we are working with and in. I offer up this section because this is the magic of a unicorn. This is where sparkle and shine emanate from — from the inside out. Wellness is about your best self; body, mind, and spirit. Weekly rituals, listed below in your weekly assignment, bring calm support and yes, more love into your life and everything you do … and that, in my (hand)book, is the healthiest thing you can do in the world — to love bigger, connect to magic, go within to shine with boundless eminence.

And let's be honest, who doesn't want to invoke a little magic with pretty crystals, essential oils, or tarot now and then?

If you already have spiritual rituals well established, YAY! Continue along your path and see if any of these speak to you to layer in. If you're brand new to ritual, WELCOME TO THE PARTY! Below are things to "do" daily or weekly to help ground and expand your inner unicorn. As always, these are offerings and how you choose to integrate or embrace them is completely up to you. Your spiritual ritual is deeply personal. Allow it to be a relationship that evolves and that you enjoy.

ASSIGNMENT 7 : SPIRITUAL RITUAL

Choose one or more of the rituals below. Go with your gut and trust your instincts. If ever there was a place for going with your feels, it's here. Exactly like the bedtime rituals, choose what speaks to you or what sounds like fun. Try not to judge. Embark as a unicorn would with a blend of intellect and intuition and see what it brings about.

Meditation

It's important to cultivate a time for quiet in your life.

You can call it an adult time-out, you can call it a breath, you can call it a mindfulness, or rewiring. You can call it *I do this so I don't lose my sh*t in the world* practice. Call it whatever you want. It's simply a matter of doing it. Meditation is powerful and true magic in what it brings about in a life when you practice it consistently.

To me, meditation is the most spiritual connection there is, however, there's science that goes along with it and if the spiritual label on it doesn't appeal to you, don't discard the idea. If centuries of practice in multiple countries isn't enough to sway you, science is finally catching up to prove its benefits.

A Harvard study via MRIs proves that consistent meditation increases gray matter in the brain within eight weeks.

Gray matter processes information in the brain and sends messages to (mainly) your central nervous system but it is also involved in muscle control, seeing, hearing, memory, emotions, speech, decision making, and self control. I think we can see how important it is.

The upswing you feel from a meditation practice isn't just emotional. It's hard, factual science that it improves self-awareness, introspection, and compassion. Harvard's study showed that daily meditation changes our brains for the better. It essentially makes you smarter and more efficient because a larger portion of your brain is activated. Meditation is exercise for your brain. Let's just say it, meditation is smart.

The concept of a meditation practice has gotten muddled. It's been sold to us as another strange aspirin to simply layer on top of any mess we may have going on in our lives. Meditation often feels like another thing to check off the list in order to have that *hip* current social media life. Sadly, it can feel like that, in reality it's not, it's the most real thing you'll ever do. Meditation doesn't have to be something else to do. It can be pleasurable and anticipated as a personal hug, or internal cup of tea that warms us and restores joy, optimism, and happiness.

Meditation has Numerous Benefits Proven by Science

Here are just a few:
- Decreased stress and anxiety, worry, loneliness, and depression;

- Improved resilience to pain and adversity;
- Increased optimism;
- Improved mood;
- Increased mental focus;
- Increased memory retention and recall;
- Help with managing ADHD;
- Increased creative thought and problem solving;
- Improved immune system and energy;
- Reduced blood pressure;
- Lessened inflammatory issues in the body;
- Reduced autoimmune disease symptoms;
- Lessened PMS;
- Slowed signs of aging; and
- Increased happiness

Start a simple meditation practice — free of expectations of what you think it is or should be. It's worth the time and effort to set a date for you to *get to know you* every week. You don't have to do it every day to gain benefits and a minimum of two minutes at a time makes positive impact.

I'm always about efficiency and bang-for-the-buck and #betterisbetter. You never start at the top of the mountain you decide to climb. Go one step at a time.

It's important to sit still. The capacity to sit, to do nothing, or to be bored seems to be reduced because of modern life and screens in all their manifestations. We are constantly in a state of poking, prodding, and being filled … rather than emptying out and allowing creativity to flow into us. Call it divine thought or inspiration, meditation is powerful magic that leads us home to ourselves and the expansive unknown of the ethers.

Meditation is the Practice of Doing Nothing

Creating space in your brain is nothing but good for you. Empty, white, quiet space allows for thoughts, answers, and ideas. A connection to your thoughts is the name of the game when it comes to meditation. It's about awareness of what's in that noggin of yours and how those thoughts influence everything you do and directly affect what manifests in your life.

It's true that you are what you eat and even truer that you experience what you think.

The biggest misconception of a meditation practice is that you must quiet your mind. The biggest excuse is "I tried meditation … but I could never *shut off* my brain." Or "I couldn't *be quiet*" or "I was too noisy … so I quit." Ummmmm ok, so we're judging our quiet time now? We're competing in our capacity to just *be*? We're farther off the radar than I had hoped. QUICK! Harness that unicorn spirit of yours and throw some glitter on that concept. Unravel those antiquated excuses and shift into the idea that if we are each divinely unique, our meditation practices can be too.

Let's be clear, humans have cognitive capacity. It's what separates us from the animals.
Our capacity to think. The goal may NOT be to be quiet, silent, still, or empty. After all, we are designed to think. Stopping that process may not be the ultimate or appropriate goal for everyone.

I invite you to think about meditation as a wonderful opportunity for active minds to simply be aware of what all those zipping thoughts are. Most of us aren't really even aware of what our heads/thoughts are filled with. Meditation is the opportunity to see what's in there.

Meditation is just like opening the attic. Or dumping out your backpack. What have you stashed in there? How often do you clean and sort it? Do you have gorgeous gems or piles of out-of-date magazines? Are you filled with useful, positive thoughts or degrading, self-abusive thinking? Are you hauling around generations of false paradigms or are you working with your own beliefs? All of this directly influences your ability to achieve your fitness, wellness, and yes, life goals.

You don't have to feel that you've already failed at some false idea of perfect, silent, yogi-on-the-mount meditation. This handbook is here to give you permission to craft your own meditation practice that is uniquely yours. Find your own way to be present to your own thoughts so you see what's really running and driving you. What ideas and voices are steering your internal ship? The biggest beautiful piece of all of this is that when you start to hear and see what internal dialogue is running, you get to craft and tweak it as you like. There's magic in the crafting.

It takes time but I can absolutely promise you that the things you're scared of knowing are far less scary once they've been seen and identified. Exactly like turning the lights on in a closet full of monsters — once the lights are on … there are no monsters.

Take some time to connect with your divine self. Take some time to cultivate your own voice, intuition, and gut instincts. Take the time to exercise your internal moral compass so you can know how you *feel* about things even when you may not really know what you think about things.

Your feels are different from your feelings. Your feels are those deep gut instincts and ultimate knowing. Your feelings are an emotional layer of being human. Both valid and real … but we want to get to the place where the feels are running the show not the feelings. Your feels are your internal compass. You know when you feel safe and happy or when things *just don't feel right*. This is your intuition. This is your truth. This is your unicorn magic.

Too much noise in your life doesn't allow space for the awareness of your feels. No empty space in your brain results in little to no internal compass, and then you set yourself up to be led by external messaging of the pixels of the world verses making choices about what you want and need for the highest and greatest good of your best self, your unicorn self.

Noise puts up blocks and shields. Empty space is where love lives. Empty space is where great ideas and real solutions come from.

You're the vessel of at least one beautiful idea that will make at least one thing in the world better. We each have a gift to give to make the world a better place. But if there's no quiet time to hear, realize, or *think up* these things … you might miss your opportunity to make a positive impact in the world. I'd hate to waste the magic of any unicorn.

But before you can throw your personal magic around you're going to need to cultivate it. It's time to see what you've got stashed in your attic. It's time to clean out the cobwebs, turn on the closet lights and emanate iridescent rainbows from the inside out.

Four simple unicorn tactics to practice meditation:

1. Listen to Binaural Beats - Binaural beats are fascinating and the most useful passive meditation you'll find. They can also be called personal hypnosis and should be listened to with headphones for optimal benefit. Binaural beats are two separate sound frequencies, one played in each ear, and your brain actually hears a third tone … the *fill in* sound. This engages the parts of the brain that cultivate calm and focus just as a seated, silent meditation practice does. Planetary frequencies and hemi syncing are my favorites in this category.
2. Go Old School - Sit in silence for two to 20 minutes at a time.
3. Vibe to Rhythms - Listen to meditative music two to 20 minutes at a time.
4. Be Guided - Do my monthly guided meditation video at www.unicornwellnessstudio.com. I

post one guided meditation every month. You can do it as often as you like in that month. It allows you to shift and engage with the collective energies of each month and go deep with that month's particular concept because what we need to balance our energies and cultivate divine connection is ever evolving with the stars, the moon, and the calendar.

Tarot and Oracle Decks

These are often unfairly misunderstood. Many still think about the tarot as fortune telling; prediction cloaked in dark arts and bad juju. Well, you probably don't because you're on the unicorn path … bless you for that but if you're somewhere in the middle or simply don't have an opinion about them at all, I'm here to offer them as a simple tool of divination.

A tool of divination is a ritual, practice, or tactic that allows you to connect with your intuition/higher self more clearly. It's also said that each and every person has a tool of divination … one that they personally connect with more than others, to assist them in their connection to divine messaging and their intuition; the ability to understand something immediately, without the need for conscious reasoning.

Other tools include meditation, runes, tea leaves, melted wax puddles, and yes crystals or crystal balls.

The Tarot

Tarot cards are much more loving, supportive, optimistic, and systematic than most people give them credit for. They're a tool for deeper thought, introspection, and self awareness. Tarot or oracle cards are a way to clear an emotional path through confusion and are far more systematic than you realize. They are my tool of choice. Or rather, the tool that chose me. I think of them as an old school landline switch-board that help plug us into our higher self in a clearer, more efficient manner. Tarot or oracle cards are a wonderful choice for those that love symbolism, myth, and metaphor. Signs, symbols, and omens are a language unto themselves and some find great comfort, ease, and talent in them while others go … 'uhhhh I have no idea what that meant.' Whichever response you have is OK. Unicorns are unique and therefore the things we attach to and connect with will be as well — except for rainbows, sparkles, glitter, all things iridescent, you know, the essentials.

To begin to work with cards, just pick a deck you like. This is extremely important. If you find the imagery and artwork on a deck interesting, it *speaks to you* and you'll be able to read, understand, and integrate the messages better.

Tarot is meant to be a point of understanding. Like a self therapy session of sorts. You can either ask a question or simply pull a card(s) of the day and see what messages they bring you. Every tarot deck (oracles decks are different and I'll explain them in a moment) comes with a booklet of meanings for that particular deck. It's as simple as playing with the deck you picked then reading the booklet to connect with them for the cards you pulled.

There is no *right* answer and when you start. It will all feel like make-believe and silliness and muckiness. The more often you pull tarot cards the easier it gets. Like anything, practice breeds mastery. I find that the usefulness of the booklets varies on a deck-to-deck basis. The booklet that comes with each deck shares that deck's particular guidelines and definitions for each card. There is a strong history of meaning in the tarot but be clear, we're working with divine energy, you're connecting to your personal intuition and the cards you choose are yours and the messages that images bring you are yours. Your personal understanding of the card will always be the *right* message.

I tend to be someone who writes their own book (see what I did there?) rather than follow one that already exists. I often bypass the booklet initially with a new deck. I love to get a feel for each deck's personality and what I get from it rather than being told what I'm *supposed* to get from it. It often takes about a month for me to make friends with my deck. It takes time to connect to the energies of each deck. Allow the time and connection to unfold. I've had decks for years that I go back to and *finally* connect with.

In my opinion, going with your gut is the true method of receiving messages via the cards, as they are a connection to your intuition. But, if your intuition needs some strengthening and it feels like more of a challenge to connect with messaging, USE THE BOOKLETS! Always go with your gut. If the meaning in the booklet rings true for your inquiry, hooray! If the booklet just doesn't feel right to you … it's not and your intuition is already working. Go, unicorn go!

Think of tarot as the exercise to strengthen your intuition muscle. Meditation strengthens the intellect and energies and allows for clearer intuitive messages but the tarot gives functional practice of sifting, sorting, and translating those messages and how to apply them in your life.

Tarot cultivates confidence in your feels — remember feels are different than your feelings. Poor little feelings may feel challenged by the cards and may have a hard time initially working with the messages, but there's gold in the growth of self love and emotional intelligence. The tarot cultivates the ability to abide by what's right for you. It allows you to initiate conversations with your heart and start to explore questions and choices at a depth you just probably won't without them. If you anchor into a card practice regularly it will strengthen the ability to take action on what is right for you — not everyone else. You'll feel more supported by the universe because there was a tangible card/message.

A tarot practice allows you to sift and sort, receive guidance then make decisions and choices based in love, well meaning, growth and solid ownership of said decisions. Eventually you'll actually make better decisions because you inquire and deeply connect to the divine via your personal intuition.

And if you're still not sold on the idea of creating a direct connection to your divine messages, guides, guardian angels, or higher self, then approach them from the placebo perspective: the cards bring up for you in the moment of the reading deserves attention, contemplation, and awareness. Simple as that. Give thought to how the stories of myths and archetypes resonate in our souls. It's important to take the time for self reflection and evaluation in respect to infinite energies and historical symbolism. The tarot is highly systematic and helps sort your feelings — yes, *those* feelings this time … the emotional, human ones that we must learn to balance — in order to anchor into, strengthen, and navigate from your feels.

The unicorn transformation comes from a balance of intellect, intuition, and love via self-care and magic. Tend to your earthy physical needs — food, water, shelter — in combination with finding balance in your feels, feelings, and analytical thinking. That's where magic lives.

Oracle Cards

These are a little different than tarot and perhaps better for beginners. Tarot has a deep system and language unto itself with the Major Arcana and all the suits of the Minor Arcana that can take a lifetime to truly *learn* (not to scare you off) but oracle cards stand alone. They are straightforward with direct phrases or quotations and come in super fun formats like guardian angels or even unicorn decks! You can work with them just as you do with the tarot, seeing what your instincts and intuition say about the card to you. What do the pictures on the cards make you think of? What do they bring to mind? What color, scent, song, person, or story does it remind you of? This is where the goods are in either type of card. Take note of what the card(s) you pull says or represents and see

what meaning it has for you in that moment. See how that thought, information or idea can benefit the situation or question you are seeking guidance on. Always look at the info in reference to the better, highest and greatest good of all involved.
Getting Started

After you've picked a deck you connect with, make sure to clear it of any energy it may have picked up on its path to you. I clear my cards just as I clear crystals: smudge them with incense, mugwort, sage, or palo santo. As you wave the smoke over and around the deck just say a little well wishes prayer out loud or in your head that sounds similar to or exactly like:

"Please allow this deck to release any and all negative energies it may have picked up on its way to me. Please restore its energies that divinity intended to bring through messages from my guides and guardian angels that I can easily understand from the highest and greatest good of all involved, rooted in love and light."

Another option is to light a candle and wave the deck above the white light with that exact or similar prayer. I tend to do both … I'm a type-A personality who loves to clean and adores ritual.

Historically you're *supposed* to store them in silk or velvet for protection. I keep mine in one of my grandmother's scarves when I travel … otherwise I just leave them sitting out with a crystal sitting on top of the deck.

It's always a good idea to connect a tarot practice with a meditation practice. It strengthens the the practice.

Card Layouts

Two card layouts I recommend starting with are; a simple Card of the Day or Past-Present-Future pull.

Start small. The Card of the Day is just as it says, shuffle and pull one a day. See what energy it and how or if it influences you and your day. Try pulling one in the morning than revisiting it at the end of your day. See if it has new meaning after the day has finished and start to see how your initial interpretations unfold within 24 hours.

In the second card layout, pull three cards and lay them in a row. Past. Present. Future. The first card will represent your past - could be yesterday, could represent years ago — only you will know, the second will represent the present energies you are working with and the third is the future — later in the day, tomorrow, end of the year — again it's about your experience and understanding of the card and what question you are seeking guidance on. The more you practice the stronger and more clear your messaging will be. As in all things, true understanding comes with time but you'll be delighted and shocked as to how such a simple act of introspection and reflection can truly start to change the quality of your life.

There are an innumerable card layouts. A little Googling will have you inundated with options. Play. Work with what speaks to you. And if you prefer supported readings from a teacher as you learn your way, you can connect with my monthly readings on www.unicornwellnessstudio.com. Pulling for yourself creates incredible connection to your unicorn nature, yet every student needs a teacher and a guide. Even the most seasoned reader will have their cards read by someone they trust to bring illuminated guidance to an inquiry.

Mala Beads

You may know them for their connection to yoga but I like to use them in day-to-day life by holding them at bedtime rather than counting sheep, or starting or ending my day. I find them a wonderful tool for calming anxiety. Simply count the beads (108) and pick one mantra to repeat: a wish, a prayer, or a calming affirmation. Say anything you wish each time you count/touch a bead. It should be affirming and positive. Short and sweet is best. For example "I sparkle and shine from the

inside out!" What you repeat enough …
you begin to believe. It's a beautiful and
simple way to program yourself for the
positive. When you first start these
practices do they feel like faking it or
pretending? Sure do. Fake it till you make
it…...as I prefer...Faith it till you make
it…have faith that you are drawn to these
practices to support and evolve to your
best self.

Repetition cultivates mastery. Unicorns
make sure what they repeat creates love,
light, and positive evolution.

Pick a set of beads that speaks to you, a
color or shape you like, that are inspiring or
comforting. Again, much of spiritual ritual is
simply about enjoying what you are doing.
Beads don't need to be fancy. A little etsy
scrolling and you'll find a wonderful piece
that bubbles up magic in you.

Crystals

Crystals have healing powers. As energy is neither created nor destroyed plus the fact that we are all made up of energy, crystals are powerful and delightful conduits of healing unicorn vibes. Every individual crystal carries a particular energy that can be harnessed and synthesized to support our divine nature. Each crystal carries a particular healing quality in their energetic field. When we hold, carry, wear, meditate or surround ourselves with, we integrate their dynamic energies into our own. They support spiritual ritual and pretty up any space they reside in. Unicorns put deep faith in the energies of the sparkle and shine of healing crystals.

Pick a stone or stones that *speak* to you. Look online, visit a local crystal and rock store, or go with my listed recommendations below.

Crystal quartz, rose quartz, agate and carnelian are wonderful *beginner* stones to work with for overall balance or grounding that don't tend to shake your energetic field too intensely initially.

I keep little piles everywhere in my home and typically have a pocketful with me wherever I go. There's nothing more complementary to a unicorn than sparkling objects!

Crystals are a bit like a grown up lovie — grounding and soothing. Their mere presence acts as a reminder of what they represent or what you'd like to work on at the time; unconditional love, calmness, deflecting negativity, transmuting negative energy to the positive etc. They help bring our humanness back into a more constructive, unicorn inhabited space.

Crystals are a welcome addition to any seated meditation practice, simply hold in your hands or lay on your body, in sleep or scattered around your tarot and oracle cards.

Pick crystals that you like. It's nice to play with them in a store so you get the tangible experience with different energies. Touch and hold each one to see what calls to you and what feels good in your hands. Ordering online works too! #betterisbetter work with what you can and don't get caught up in doing things perfectly.

Crystals offer a major opportunity to work with your intuition. Picking stones by color or look is always fun because when you look up the meaning and find it beyond appropriate for your life circumstances at the time. There are wonderful books for healing crystal meanings. You can look up the meaning you wish to work with or go with what calls to you, then look up its meaning after to see if it rings true for you. Take the route that feels best for you. But have no fear, I've got some unicorn recommendations for you as well.

Caring for your Crystals

Each time you get a new crystal you'll need to cleanse it of any negative energies it may have absorbed prior to arriving in your care. 'Cause it did its job and pulled negative energies out of whatever environment they were in prior to making its way to you.

Cleansing your Crystals

Smudge each crystal with incense, mugwort, sage, or palo santo. Waft the smoke over and around the crystals while saying a small prayer out loud or in your head to the effect of "Release any negative energies these crystals may have absorbed and allow them to return to their original frequencies as mother nature intended to assist in my healing and protection."

You can also program crystals for something specific you are working on improving in your life. It's not necessary to program your crystals, but if you have a clear goal that you want intense and direct assistance releasing or transmuting, a little extra energy in that direction won't hurt. For example, if the issue you are trying to evolve from is undeservedness or unworthiness or releasing a bad habit, you program the crystal by saying a prayer, out loud or to yourself, to the effect of "Please assist me in embracing and honoring my full self worth. I am worthy." or "Please assist me in releasing the habit of gossiping. I only participate in constructive dialogue." Then you're ready to roll.

It's also important to recharge your stones during the Full Moon every month. Look up when the moon cycles are. On the night of the full moon — or up to two days before and after — smudge all your stones with the same tools you originally cleansed them with, say your cleansing prayer as you did above, then set all your stones outside in the moonlight or in a window sill near the full moon for 24 hours.

Crystals work based on energies. They balance and uplift energetic fields. Crystals absorb negative elements to leave you with positive ones. They work hard for us, so they need to release that negative energy … otherwise that negative energy gets carried and passed around or blocks the crystal from doing its positive balancing work.

At its most intense, negative energy that becomes too much for a crystal will break or shatter the piece. Dramatic as it may seem I've witnessed it countless times. It's always a sign of protection and of doing its job in a big way. If you ever have a broken piece, thank it for it's hard work than bury the pieces in a plant or dirt. Return it to mother earth with a blessing. Crystals can also *get lost* when they have done their job for you.

Crystals have a divine mission of their own and can find their way to or away from you. Always honor that whichever journey your crystals take it is always best. As in our life journey, everything is happening as it should.

Boost your Unicorn Vibes

Healing crystals help amplify energies and, more importantly, they heal. Everyone requires healing. Healing is what our human experience is all about. If you connect with and pick the right crystals they can be a sparkling and shining way to do just that. If you're not already a crystal-toting moon momma think of them as little flashlights that point to certain things in the world like love, confidence, abundance, healing deep wounds, etc. They bump off the energy to certain things ... just like essential oils … there's a crystal for that! You can set them out among your ritual, wear them or tuck them in your pockets.

1. **Pink Banded Agate** - These hot pink beauties scream fun, while balancing yin and yang promotes a fierce femme vibe in the wearer. This stone promotes love in an unabashed way. Agate in general is earthy, rooted, and grounding. Pink banded agate soothes anger, transmutes negativity, and protects and cleanses your aura. It's a #loveoutloud #feircelove kinda stone.

2. **Pearl** - The pearl is a sneaky siren of the sea that is drastically overlooked when it comes to healing

crystals. It's long been touted as a symbol of femininity that helps cultivate your inner goddess and because it comes from the ocean is directly connected to lunar energies, feminine energies, the energy of intuition, and psychic abilities. It supports your inner truth, personal integrity, and allows us to open up to our true selves in a soothing and calm way. Pearls are the divine feminine energy at it's best — mysterious, powerful, understated yet glamorous and calm.

3. **Rainbow Aura Quartz** - The next two crystals, in my opinion, are the most unicorn in nature. Rainbow Aura Quartz is quartz crystal that has been treated with titanium and gold. You heard me, the strongest and one of the world's most treasured metals combined with the magic of crystal. Typically I'm a purist. I don't like things messed with by man, but I feel like this one is the internet of woowoo magic. It's rooted in a genuine connection to mother earth with a

modern tech spin. This crystal comes out looking like a black iridescent rainbow. This crystal called to me for months. In dreams, in my Facebook feed, and in my local shops, it even arrived in the mail as a gift. Yup, my guides are clear and persistent. It carries a super metallic vibe like the buzzing superconductor of crystals. This stone carries more yang, masculine, energy that cultivates a zest for life and real deal manifestation. It helps to release resentment and grief, aides in releasing karmic ties - which you need to do - in order to manifest. It's a master healer of any body disease and is excellent at healing trauma or hurt. Remember that witches wear black, not because of connection to evil spirits, but because the color deflects negativity.

4. **Opal Aura Quartz** - This one is sometimes referred to as Angel Aura quartz, but I want to rename is Unicorn Quartz. There's no reason to beat around the bush. This crystal is

the yin to Rainbow Aura Quartz's yang. This is quartz crystal that has been treated with Platinum and it comes out looking like an white iridescent rainbow. Opal Aura Quartz is the crystal of joy, hope, and optimism. It cleanses, balances, and stimulates all chakras and integrates the light body (the light body is a bit tricky to explain in absolutes but essentially it's the energetic vehicle that allows our human energy to return to divine energy). Opal Aura Quartz aims to cultivate complete union with the Divine. It's pure magic in a rainbow crystal.

5.   **Amethyst** - Another multitasker this crystal is known as the *all healer*. Amethyst is known to be the healer's stone to cure all that ails you. It's a natural tranquilizer, protective, sobering, and associated with the Temperance card in the tarot to teach and cultivate balance in all areas of your life. Amethyst is also connected to the Seventh Chakra, your crown chakra, the receiver of divine

messages. It heightens intuition and psychic abilities because of its connection to the direct messaging of Spirit. It aids in reprogramming negative paradigms and assists in positive self talk. Its hallmarks are creativity and spirituality.

6.   **Black Tourmaline -** Is also known as schorl and is a personal favorite of mine. All black stones are excellent for grounding (basically, helping to assuage anxiety and fear) they also deflect negative vibes but this one actually transmutes any negative vibes it encounters and transmutes them into positive vibes! What?! Layers of magic here. You can see how it's great to have near your full moon rituals of releasing.

7.   **Smoky Quartz -** Smoky quartz is a more traditional stone of protection against negative energy but it's got the bonus of pulling out blocks you may not even know about from deep inside you, to assist in the process of release and forgiveness and integrating your shadow side. It's a

great one for those who aren't sure what isn't working or have energetic blocks you haven't identified yet. They are powerful transformers and not for the faint of heart. They can bring up major hurts, but this signals the ignition of healing. Be gentle with the process and honor its strength.

8. **Jade** - Jade comes in many colors, each with its own variation on its meaning but overall Jade is a tender, subtle stone of self love, protection, and luck with a sweetness and lightness that screams unicorn nature. My favorite Jades are turquoise - for serenity, pink - for wise grandmotherly love, sea mist green - luck, and lavender - for spiritual nourishment.

9. **Moonstone** - Clearly its name would be enough as to why it made the list but there's more to it than that. It's more aligned with the new moon as a stone of new beginnings but it's truly 50/50 for new and full moon. It's said to soothe emotional instability and amplify intuition. The moon is

about all the unseen information, intuition, and psychic connection. Whatever you want to call it, this stone amplifies it. It's connected to the element of water; the 3rd and 6th chakra; manifesting and intuition. It's utterly feminine and anchored in the goddess energy. I wear moonstone daily.

10. **Rose Quartz -** Rose quartz amplifies love, opens and heals the energy of the heart. It makes you more receptive to love and more capable of giving love without depleting your energy as it knows the karmic law of 'what you reap you sow' when giving love is practiced with true intention. Rose quartz is associated with the heart chakra. Love is the only true and ultimate energy. It is the energy of divine spirit. Love heals all, it's the only true answer for all problems. Rose quartz is a gentle and sweet cure all.

11. **Selenite -** Selenite is named for the Greek word 'Selene' meaning moon. It's white and satiny and luminous.

It's a healing crystal said to integrate your ethereal (light) and physical bodies. The *light body* we spoke of earlier loves this stone. It heals and amplifies your intuition. It's a stone of clarity. It helps clarify your thoughts to strengthen your ability to make decisions you're confident in. This is a super sweet, calm and gentle way to assist your confidence and making, as well as executing, decisions. It's a stone of intuition whose energy is directly linked to the energy of the moon. It's wonderful for women to help sync their feminine cycle to the new moon cycle for deep rooted momma earth connection and hormone balance.

Essential Oils

Essential Oils, or EO's as there are often referred to, are natural oils typically obtained by distillation from plants. The oils that are produced in distillation contain the *essence* of each plant's healing properties and scent.

Essential oils have been used medicinally and aromatically for centuries. I believe all things momma earth creates are far superior and safer than the majority of man-made substances, I'm a firm advocate for essential oils for supporting the invocation and sustainability of all unicorns. EO's bridge the functional and ethereal spaces in this earthly plane.

EO's can cover the basics, from killing bacteria and fungus to soothing an achy tummy to healing skin issues at an accelerated rate. They also offer up energetic and emotional support via aromatherapy.

The list below are the essential EO's for unicorns.

Unicorns tend to be super sensitive, utterly empathetic, supreme do-ers, and real deal work horses in the giving and care-of-others department which can often leave them depleted, anxious, nervous, or simply tired. All of the essential oil recommendations below support, protect, and balance these issues.

Toss a few drops of high grade, preferably organic, essential oils on your pillow at night or to a bath. Simply slather on your wrists, hands and feet, forearms and chest to breathe in and reap the rewards of their magic. You're always welcome to use a carrier oil with your oils, such as; sesame oil, olive oil or fractionated coconut oil but none of the essential oils on our unicorn list are caustic enough to require a carrier. I just slather them on my skin when I need a little extra sparkle support.

Bolster and balance your unicorn vibes with these Essential Oils:

1. **Frankincense** - Frankincense offers us support in our capacity to focus our spiritual awareness. It aids in translating the signs, symbols, and omens that appear in our lives from

divine spirit. It's grounding and earthy and helps us integrate our higher selves into our day-to-day. It also relieves tension, stress, and anxiety. It calms a nervous system and supports our overall energy and life force. If you only work with one essential oil, this is the ultimate unicorn elixir.

2. **Lavender** - This one is probably the most well known essential oil of them all and many of you are cringing at it being highlighted. What could be more *basic (read as non-magical)* than lavender? If you're like I used to be, you've only experienced low grade lavender that smells like cheap soap and has you repelling at the thought of adding it to your days. When it comes to lavender you've got to go high grade on the oil source,

you simply can't buy cheap. When you experience a high end oil you'll see what all the fuss is about. It's dreamy and yes, assists with slumber. Lavender is calming, relaxing, antibacterial, antiseptic, anti-inflammatory, and an antidepressant. Its main benefit is helping to maintain a healthy nervous system, which allows for more patience, more calm, better focus, and better presence. It's a wonderful sleep aid because of its capacity to down regulate your sympathetic nervous system. Sprinkle a few drops of this one on your pillow prior to bedtime or make a spritzer out of it with 8 oz. of distilled water plus five to 15 drops of lavender essential oil and spray yourself and your sleeping area about 20 minutes prior to rest.

3. **Rose** - Just like rose quartz is the ultimate healing crystal and carries the vibration of love, rose essential oil is the ultimate uplifting healer when it comes to EO's. Rose is love. Love is the ultimate energy and the ultimate healer. Rose can be challenging to come by in a cost effective option because it's the real deal carrier of magical feminine, nurturing love. It's also a soothing anti-depressant, anti-inflammatory, antiviral that protects plus increases cell growth to assist in functional healing, self-esteem, and self-confidence. Our grandmothers had the right idea when it comes to lavender and rose for our daily scents. Go for the highest quality you can, the scents can vary greatly because of the quality and type of rose it's sourced from. Search and

sniff until your unicorn snout is happy
with a rose scent. Anything rose is a
unicorn's BFF.

4. **Ylang Ylang** - This essential oil
   supports the solar plexus, our hot
   spot for manifestation. Ylang ylang
   boosts energy, moods and supports
   a healthy digestive and reproductive
   system. It allows you to *digest* and
   stomach more of life while cultivating
   confidence and self-reliance. A few
   drops rubbed on your belly during the
   week or even daily truly works magic
   and supports your capacity to show
   up and *do* in the world.

5. **Lime** - Lime is an unsung hero of
   essential oils. It's protective, loving,
   balancing, and energizing. It
   cleanses your digestive system along
   with your spirit to allow for renewed
   infusions of a *clean slate* to work

from. Lime cools and balances a body. It's wonderful to use in the evening to wash away the day and put things to rest both on the inside and out. I add a couple of drops to a 12-oz. glass of water most evenings.

6. **Vanilla** - Vanilla is soothing scent that harkens us back to our childlike wonder with the sweet scent of baked goods. It's comforting and playful all at the same time. Because of it's relaxing nature it assists with calming hyperactivity, digestive distress and with its anti-inflammatory, antidepressant, antioxidant properties it's helpful with lowering all general stress levels.

7. **Vetiver** - Think of vetiver as an amped up patchouli. Though this oil is sourced from a grass plant it functions much more like a strong

rooted tree. It's sticky sap-like consistency is liquid gold when it comes to grounding. It's earthy, soothing, and protective. Vetiver is considered the oil of tranquility and is an excellent resource to head-off or balance exhaustion, frazzled nerves, and anxiety.

And just like a fist full of glitter being thrown your way, you've completed The Unicorn Wellness Handbook!

Bravo! As in all great mythology there is never truly an ending. An ending is just the beginning of the next chapter. These sparkle and shine tactics make life healthier, more efficient, and fun. They connect you to the divine nature we are all born with but must return to in order to truly show up in the world as our best selves. These tactics allow you to work your magic on your own time, in real time. These tactics generate unicorns that literally change the world for the better, simply by existing.

This handbook allows you to feel capable, unique, and empowered everyday. Being a unicorn is a living practice. Being a unicorn is, ironically, very real. Simply completing your handbook does not mean the work is done. Unicorns don't just mosey off into the forest to never come back again. You must continue to practice these methods, everyday, every week, and every year. It's most important to practice them when you don't feel like it, when the world seems big and scary, toxic and overwhelming. Putting your unicorn practices into actual practice is where the true magic is.

Our human life is all about allowing the divine spirit to show up here, in real time. Our tests, lessons, trials, roadblocks, and hiccups are all opportunities to show our guides, guardian angels, higher self, and God that we're willing to put the work in. All the lessons are about showing how responsible we can and will be when our true wishes, wants, and manifestations finally arrive. Yes, the hard times are tests. But guess what? As in all tests, the more you study the easier they get. Because you are more capable at handling, solving, answering, and working with them rather than being blown to emotional, psychological, or actual physical smithereens.

Remember that if you are an empath, highly sensitive, an introvert, have autoimmune issues, or are HUMAN you are also a unicorn. It's your birthright to sparkle and shine. You just need to know the actual steps to take in order to harness your inner unicorn … and here they are.

As Anne Morrow Lindbergh wrote in 'The Unicorn'

"He could leap the corral,
If he rose
To his full white height;
He could splinter the fencing light,
With three blows
Of his porcelain hoofs in flight —
If he chose.

He could shatter his prison wall,
Could escape them all —
If he rose,
If he chose."

Becoming a unicorn is a choice that requires repetition and will never be without mishaps, trip-ups, or mistakes. Becoming a unicorn is about the doing. Showing up and stepping outside of your comfort zone and allows you to jump your personal corral.

Becoming a unicorn is about answering the call of the unicorn.

Which you have. Which you did. Which you are — simply by reading The Unicorn Wellness Handbook.

Being a unicorn is all about how you navigate, where your intention is and the belief that magic and infinite possibilities exist … *and that **you** are that magic and possibility.*

HOW TO NOURISH A UNICORN

Unicorns need to be nourished with great care. They are sensitive and magical. They straddle the physical and spiritual realms and this requires a delicate balance of fuel. Unicorns require their nourishment to be pristine and clean, steeped in pleasure to love on them from the inside out, literally. Unicorns are a unique tribe that do things their own way. They never follow the herd of mundane horses. They seek out the real, genuine foods that allow them to heal and thrive … leaving behind the dark gray vibes of mere survival.

Cracking your personal food code via my 41 Day Food Reset invokes your inner unicorn at a powerful cellular level. Cracking your personal food code will have you radiating rainbow energy on every level.

The Reset

It's time to crack your personal food code.

My food philosophy is simple: **KEEP. IT. REAL.** As a unicorn I'm a purist at heart. I want the real deal of everything. I want high quality without being wasteful and I want things as momma earth intended them to be that work in harmony with our bodies rather than against them. Our bodies are designed beautifully. They are perfect the moment we are born but the external forces of a concrete world laden with pixels, products, and synthetics make that perfection challenging to reign supreme.

We need to be more diligent, in this day and age, about how we feed our bodies. We're seeing obesity, autoimmune, and metabolic issues at a rate we've never seen before. Much of this comes from not living in accordance with how our bodies are designed to thrive — on whole real foods, with spiritual ritual, calm movement, hydration … as a unicorn. The buildup of GMOs, pesticides, nitrates, antibiotics, and generations of chemically laden soil sources that our food is treated with and grown in has created hurdles to health life never before.

Food is the greatest medicine.
We are what we eat.
Food can either be our greatest healer or our slowest killer.

The cliches are true.

The beautiful part of this is that our health and wellness problems are solved and made better in such a simple and pleasurable way … THROUGH OUR FOOD! Cracking your own food code gives you the keys to your personal kingdom. It's about what works for you — now, at this current age and stage in your life — without judgment, without abiding by someone else's comforts or limitations. It's about your best self, by you, for you.

When we up the quality of the foods we eat we say yes, yes, YES to our birthright of a healthy body that sings with happiness and energy!

Real always wins when it comes to health and wellness, but that being said, the exact details of the foods that generate healing and radiate energy for each person is *slightly* different. Bodies are wise and they know what works. Your body is trying to tell you right now what's not working. It talks to you day-after-day, year-after-year. Cravings and imbalances are real … it's our translation and reactions that are off. The Reset teaches you how to navigate the call and response of your own body. These 41 days cultivate a conversation between body and food that does nothing but get better over time.

The goal of the Reset is to figure out what foods help your body to realize vibrant health and vitality from the inside out. The Reset allows your gut to take a break from the toxins found in chemically laden, pre-packaged, and processed foods and helps to identify what does and does not work for your body at this point in time. Every-body is a little different. And although real foods always work, even some of them can trip up our bodies on our path to fitness and wellness results. The Reset lays the groundwork for true gut health that leads you to long-term fitness and wellness results. The 41 days you spend exploring your personal food adventure is a chance to connect to your food from a perspective of healing and fueling rather than one of:

1. Ignorance — Because not knowing or not understanding how a body and food work together is real and the Reset educates you in a way nothing else has.

2. Emotional Comfort — This is probably the biggest hurdle to your best health. As humans we get so stuck in what is easy or what everyone else is doing or the fear of not wanting to be wrong about what we've eaten. We hate transitions and challenges, all the while knowing that doing the harder things are often the most powerful and important. Emotional comfort is limiting and sheltering. It's stunting to a soul and to your health.

3. Entertainment and Convenience —
These are huge. We have become a
culture of thinking that eating should be
fun, fast, and entertaining at all times,
losing complete track of the fact that food is
a tool of our survival and thrival. Eating
purely from an entertainment perspective is
dangerous. Inside the entertainment we
distance ourselves from thinking, doing,
and creating. We see it as something that
should always be pleasing or of one-upping
the last meal. Eating for entertainment or
convenience becomes an addiction
because we're more focused on the picture
of it we took or the story we can tell about it
rather than how we feel after we ate it or
how it nurtured, supported or bolstered us.

Too many of us don't get #inthekitchen
because of our concepts of food
emotionally or functionally. Because of our
busy lives and the easy availability of pre-
cooked, packaged foods and restaurants
we have generations that don't know how
to really cook. I know, because I was one
of them. It can be scary to craft a meal from
your own two hands but it's also

unbelievably empowering! The Reset teaches you to prep and batch cook in order to efficiently live a healthy and fit lifestyle — actually taking the stress out of your meals rather than adding to your already long to-do list. Connecting with your food generates great pleasure in your life once you learn how. Cooking with love and intention is a powerful experience. Learning how to prep and cook your own meals doesn't have to be intimidating … you don't have to become a master chef or a *foodie* to connect with your meals. You just have to want to try and see what it's like and the impact it can have on the overall quality of your life. You simply need to give it a fair try.

We are What We Eat

Everything that you consume eventually shows up in or on your system, i.e. low energy levels, mood swings, eczema, acne, additional weight, bloating, gas, headaches, heartburn, those pesky little bumps on the back of your arm that everyone keeps telling you to just exfoliate more to rid yourself of. Your body can be healthy and have very few issues, great sleep and tons of energy if you fuel and treat it well. Food is a much larger part of the puzzle than you realize. If you reset your internal systems (digestion, excretion, endocrine, taste buds etc.), then you can reach optimal health with everything chugging along as it should — eating, breaking down elements, absorbing nutrients, and releasing what you do not need. It's pretty simple, what you *wear* on the inside of your body is what you *wear* on the outside as well.

Reset your Body and Heal your Gut

Getting your body from where it is to where you want it to be requires resetting and healing. Your gut needs a little down time periodically, just like your computer does. Your body deserves a break from the crazy chemicals, hormones, additives, and food products that take an incredible amount of work for your system to digest. By taking out the synthetic flavors, high doses of sugar, HFCS, and all-around harsh ingredients you consume, you allow your taste buds to actually change and … reset. You will actually begin to crave real, fresh veggies and fruit rather than being held hostage and literally addicted to fake sugars and chemicals.

By embarking on the Reset you let your digestive system physically take a rest and you give your gut — stomach, small and large intestines, liver, gallbladder, and pancreas — time to heal from any damage caused by eating foods that are not a fit for your system. Unless you are in literal perfect health, you've got at least one these not-a-fit-for-us-foods in your current fuel rotation. They cause bloating, constipation, diarrhea, acne, anxiety, difficulty concentrating, fatigue, insomnia, and even depression. You don't need to be allergic to a food to have an issue with it. Your ill-at-ease or out-of-balance symptoms don't have to be drastic or need to be medically diagnosed in order to be real or affecting your body and general quality of life. For those of us with major diagnosed autoimmune issues like IBS, Celiac, Hashimoto's Disease, Hypothyroidism, Fibromyalgia, thyroiditis, thyroidectomy, psoriasis, arthritis, eczema, or Raynaud's — just to name a few — cracking our personal food code is the lynchpin to our wellness and upswings. Healing and sealing the gut allows your body to function in the way it's created to. It will absorb more nutrients, flush and metabolize faster, and no longer have to work against all the toxins in the standard American diet or fire our autoimmune system to be in constant distress mode. In other words, it will be healthy.

In order to reset and heal your body and allow the optimal version of yourself to emerge, you must cook more. Cooking with love is a real thing and it's the only way we really know what's in our food. I teach clients to connect at your core on all levels — the core of your physical body, the core of your workouts, the core of your wellness beliefs, the core of your spirit and the core of your food. A damaged gut flat out prevents the best efforts of fitness and wellness results. This includes weight loss … not simply the big scary autoimmune issues I listed prior. Like it or not, if you want results from your body, you'll need to address your gut and crack your own food code.

Why Do We Need to Heal our Gut?

Toxins and diets with an overload of difficult to digest foods cause actual damage to your digestive system that include tears and holes in the organ tissue as well as smashed villi in your intestines that cause malabsorption of nutrients. If your guts are "leaky" or damaged they cannot absorb or process nutrients properly. Damaged guts cause hormone imbalance and lead to metabolic disorders and ease of weight loss or weight gain. A damaged gut makes everything in the realm of wellness harder because the body cannot get what it needs (nutrients) to functionally repair or thrive. Plain and simple — your body will not get what it needs from your food if you don't allow your gut to heal. Malabsorption of nutrients can lead to malnutrition and malnutrition takes you down a path of chronic illnesses, weak immune systems, potentially triggering major diseases and disorders and poor health in general. Gut damage can include but is not limited to basic *grumpy* bellies that are gassy, crampy, or distressed by chronic constipation or diarrhea, autoimmune disorders, Type -2 diabetes, chronic cystic acne, brain fog or feeling like there's a *scrim* between you and the rest of the world, finding it super hard to concentrate, short term memory issues, and heart disease.

Each body requires something different in order to thrive. For some it's clean animal protein, for others vegan is the way to go. Others exclude all grains or nightshades from their diets to allow their system to thrive. To figure out what works for your body you have to take the time to strip things out to begin with a clear baseline then reintroduce categories of foods back in one at a time and take notes on how your body responds. Your body knows itself best. You can follow diets and protocols for years but until you take the time to reset and learn what actually works for your individual body, you will never truly know what allows you to thrive.

During the Reset you will learn how to connect and listen to your body. Your body talks to you, but often the message is lost in translation. By the end of the Reset you will have cracked your own food code.

During the 41 days you'll eat veggies, fruits, good fats, probiotics, and clean, lean animal protein.

Note of Interest

I absolutely support, respect, and understand the choice of being vegan from a moral perspective as well as an environmental perspective, however there is not a vegan option for the Reset.

The Reset is written from a gut healing perspective and the only proven method to repair the organ tissues after they have been damaged is to heal and seal with collagen from clean animal protein.

If you are already thriving with a vegan diet and know that it is your personal food code, yay! Much love and wellness to you — you have no need for the Reset.

However, if you are indeed struggling with your personal best health and wellness and are seeking answers, results and upswings you'll need to consider the Reset from a perspective of medicine/healing via food. Food is an incredible healer.

I have clients who come from a vegan lifestyle and anchor into deep meditation and come around to the Reset for healing purposes while others, from the moral perspective of a vegan lifestyle simply can't make the leap to the Reset. Some choose to honor animals above their personal health, some honor their personal wellness and thank the animals for their gift of self in their journey to thrival. I respect and honor both.

Some bodies do not thrive on a vegan diet, regardless of gut damage. Some temperaments and constitutions require a bit of clean animal protein to fully thrive. I am one of those bodies. I have attempted to live vegan many times, because of the environmental and moral component. My system fails, in a huge way and this is not an uncommon experience. My experiences of eating vegan many, many times is a major part of what led me to write the Reset.

Much of our understanding of health and wellness comes from PR and marketing or self-opinions/belief minus broad research and without exploring and figuring out how our own personal systems work. I lived under the impression for years that to be as healthy as possible, I *needed* to be 100% plant based. When it comes to food/fuel, your personal food code varies depending on the body. It's important that we learn to honor how our personal systems react and respond to things vs. what we are told or think *should* work or *is best.*

The Reset is healing, and the majority of bodies that I have trained in the last two decades have gut damage to some extent regardless of medical diagnosis. This is due to the fact that gut damage has to be so extreme in order to get a positive diagnosis that most people can't get medical confirmation for an average of nine to 12 years. Our intestines/guts are 23 feet long, they require 75% damage before tests show affirmative results. A body can experience all the pain and symptoms of the damage the entire time prior to diagnosis … meanwhile people are living in unwell bodies but coming up empty handed on positive test results. This is not only in reference to digestive disorders. Gut damage also contributes to anxiety, depression, weight gain or loss that will not budge, eczema, psoriasis, acne, and bloating.

The reality of our food sources is that for generations now, the soil they are grown in has been pumped with chemicals and antibiotics. These toxins are absorbed into the crops grown in that soil, then consumed by us. These practices of non-organic farming have been and are causing massive metabolic issues at rates we've never seen in generations prior. These issues are coming from our food and we need to not only address the food, it's source, but also the healing to the intestinal and stomach lining that allows us to absorb and retain nutrients and therefore thrive.

There is a method to healing gut tissue and addressing your wellness from the inside out.

When the tears and holes in our digestive system heal, our bodies are then, and only then, capable of pulling out, absorbing, and using nutrients to thrive. The Reset addresses gut healing step-by-step in a more accessible and efficient way than other variations you may come across.

Although the statistics vary on what exact percentage of the world's population has gut damage, or leaky gut as it's often called, the numbers span from 50 to 80% of our total population. That's a lot of uncomfortable, unhealthy people that can find food-based healing that will never be found in a chemical medication! Gut tissues heal and seal via collagen from clean animal proteins, or more specifically from their bones. Collagen is the element that actually fills in the damage, hence why you cannot address gut healing from a vegan perspective.

I continually have the pleasure of witnessing the Reset invoke health upswings, major wellness turnarounds, and healing. I believe strongly in our body's innate ability to heal when given the correct, natural support to do so.

I teach a plant-based method of wellness but plant-based is not the same as vegan. Vegan is a 100% plant diet whereas plant-based means that you eat 85% to 95%

plant-based meals. This can include clean animal proteins.

If you have come to this section thinking that the only way to truly be healthy is from a completely vegan or vegetarian perspective. I ask you to expand your assumptions and approach the Reset through curiosity rather than judgment. I ask that you entertain that adding clean animal proteins to your diet, in general or strictly for healing purposes, doesn't have to mean it's a copious amount. A little truly goes a long way. It may be more in the beginning stages of healing, as it was in my experience, but as a body heals you can gradually wean it down and perhaps, for some bodies, take it out of your fuel in the long run, if your system says that it thrives best minus clean animal protein.

What Constitutes Clean and Kind Animal Proteins?

In my book a *clean* animal protein means it was wild caught or pasture raised. They are hormone-, antibiotic-, heavy metal-, chemical-, and flavoring-free. They are absolutely not processed in a factory, are organic and 100% grass-fed or when it comes to fish, not farm raised (where they are typically corn fed). Clean animal protein means they are treated with respect to their nature, fed accordingly, and given plenty of space to move freely.

Fish are not meant to consume corn and grains … where would these be found in their natural environment? But this is what they are typically fed when farm raised. Farm-raised fish are also pumped with antibiotics because the tiny environments they are raised in and are packed with bacteria. When it comes to cows, their stomachs are not built to digest grain, they are designed to eat grass … yet, mass-produced cattle are pumped with grains, antibiotics, and hormones and non-pasture raised chickens are packed into small, dark, unclean spaces.

We truly are what we eat and take on the energetics of what we consume.

Clean animal proteins matter big time. Now more than ever because we are ingesting what they have been treated with … for generations. The layers of toxins our systems are dealing with is deep and real. The cleaner the food source, the more powerful the nutrients. Dirty (conventional and factory-processed meats) are toxic, filled with chemicals and elements that are showing clear effect on our physical systems and overall health as a culture.

Eating real means having balance and respect for all of the food sources that are a fit for your personal system. If your unique body thrives with animal protein, keep it clean and keep it in balanced and minimal with respect to the amount of vegetables you're consuming.

By making clean choices in our animal proteins we are also making the most humane choice for the animal themselves, honoring their sacrifice, the cycles of life our personal health.

You don't need a lot of clean animal protein. With all foods, the cleaner it is, the least amount of processing it endures, the better it is for you and the more nutritional elements it retains. Clean foods satiate the needs of your body. Meaning, when you eat real, you don't need as much of it because it's fulfilling the true nutrient purpose of food for your body. If you're going to eat animal protein, eat clean proteins and eat smaller portions. #betterisbetter

Again, the Reset perspective is all about a wellness journey and a food adventure that is taken at face value, in the present time, day-to-day, and not colored by past experiences or perceived expectations, morality, intellectualized, emotional or false paradigms. Bodies all come from different ages, stages, experiences, toxins, diseases, and medications. The layers of a body are beautiful and even mysterious. As always, I teach what I know to be helpful, efficient and a courier of abundant wellness to as many as possible.

Is the Reset right for everyone? Nope. Does that make it *wrong*? Not at all. It simply illustrates the beauty and diversity of life.

When I speak of food in the realm of health I do so in the name of healing and not in moral or personal judgment. Wellness looks like a lot of things to a lot of people and I hold space for it all. I don't do absolutes because I know from experience that what works for a body at one point in time may very well not work at another and to be truly healthy we need to be in conversation and connection with what our bodies need and be willing to explore and respond with intelligence and care rather than react from outdated, false, emotional beliefs or simple resistance to change or the fear of *being wrong*.

Our bodies evolve every single day of our lives. They are a valuable resource that speaks to us and tell us what's not working and what it needs, we typically just have the translations wrong. the Reset allows you to learn the language of your own body. If you listen to it and abide by it, in all its evolutions and revolutions around the sun, you will heal and thrive.

Elements are not typically interchangeable. The Reset is meant to be done *as written* without swaps. I wrote it with great care, attention, and research down to cooking and prep methods. Please allow it its highest capacity of success by following it as written.

My goal is never to create or pick *sides* when it comes to food. My intention is to educate and allow you to make informed choices as to what works best for you, your food adventure, and your path to wellness.

Every body is uniquely beautiful and inherently different in the details that allow it to thrive. There are *better* choices for all bodies and there are rails in which to run for specific healing and results. However, there is not an absolute *single best* answer for all. I completely support the alkalization perspective of a vegan diet, but this not the conversations we are having when it comes to the Reset.

The Reset is written to heal your gut and crack your food code. If that works for you, HOORAY! Proceed to the kitchen. If not, that's ok! Everyone has the power of choice. Do what speaks to you and resonates in your gut ← See what I did there?

The Reset maps specific meals for five days and excludes gluten, dairy, grain, eggs, nuts, seeds, caffeine, alcohol, chocolate, nightshades, and legumes. The Reset begins with an elimination process. This is the best known way to truly identify what works for your personal system and what does not.

The five-day menu is repeated for the 41 days. This repetitive menu is your home base and will give you clear answers as to what does and does not work for you as you add in foods from your "No" list (below).

At first glance the Reset may seem highly restrictive, however the truth is, it's highly simplified to get results. By keeping the same basic five-day menu you gain mastery over your batch cooking so it can become second nature by the time you finish. Think of your Reset menu as your *control group* for your personal food experiment. By following exactly what I've written, no swaps, no modifications, etc. you allow me to guide you through your journey and you allow yourself the best possible setup for healing and clear answers for your personal food code. The repetitive menu allows for less waste, less frustration, more efficiency and clarity, less confusion, and tons of nutrient nourishment! Plain and simple, the Reset, as written, works.

An Exception to Every Rule

If you already know you are allergic to, highly sensitive to, or have major issue with certain foods simply leave them off of your personal Reset. If you have clear confirmation on things that already do not work for you there's no need to set your body back by testing them. For those with allergies or Celiac, in particular, when you get to the "add in" day for these simply take a pause, do NOT re-enter these into your food and simply wait the three to four days before going to your next add-in. The timing of when foods come back into your system matters, so please honor it and don't try to speed up your reentry process.

How the Reset Works

Certain foods are eliminated for the first five days of the Reset then layered back into your meals, one at a time, on days six through 41. All of these foods can cause difficulty to your optimal health and body over time. Just like your workouts #onthemat with me, balance is best #inthekitchen. By removing these elements for a period of time you allow your body to rest, recover, and begin to repair.

The elimination process is powerful because it clears your body and allows you to hear, see, and understand the messaging your system gives you when you eat.

Our bodies communicate with us and cravings are real. But as I've said prior, our translations and understanding of what our bodies are trying to tell us is typically way off. The Reset allows you time to learn how to communicate with your system for your optimal wellness.

The Reset is written to give you the highest amount of nourishment and bolstering in the shortest amount of time. Healing can't be hurried but I do want you to feel better as soon as possible. Trust the process. Know that the Reset literally saved my life and continues to do so. I was in continual health decline until I wrote and followed my own advice. It has also proven to save others from the pains, medications, endless doctor visits, and general problems of eating outside of their personal food code.

IBS, acne, chronic bloating, chronic constipation, diarrhea, anxiety, depression, insomnia, ADHD, ADD, migraines, headaches, psoriasis, eczema — these are just a few of the issues that have drastically improved or gone away for those who have completed the Reset and continue to abide by their personal food code. There is true power in the healing medicine of your own food code. It's time to harness it and apply it to your own body.

Also know that those of us who embark on the Reset often do so at least three times. Why? Because learning your body is a process and quite frankly, abiding by your own food code, once you've figured it out, takes practice.

The Reset is a wonderful way to heal but it's also just a wonderful home base for whole food eating and batch cooking. It takes time to really understand the power of food and getting to understand the language of your own body (what issues crop up with what foods, etc.) is truly an adventure of its own.

If you don't complete the Reset the first time, it's ok! You can do it as many times as you want or need. Every time you read it or do it you learn something new and empowering about food and yourself. It's always a worthwhile effort to embark on it.

If at any point you'd like more personalized support through your Reset process please request to join the private Facebook group The Reset to connect with those who have already or are currently completing their Reset. The group is an incredible resource for questions, comments, support, and motivation. You need to be an active www.unicornwellnessstudio.com member in order to be approved into the group.

The 'No' List

Gluten & Dairy

Gluten and dairy are the most inflammatory foods for our systems. They create swelling, bloating, and actual heat in our bodies. When you take them out you eliminate swelling, bloating, and *fire* in your system, you have less risk of infection and clear out the breeding ground for many illnesses and syndromes — the most common being cancer or autoimmune issues. With little to no inflammation, your immune system is not on constant alert. Your body finally gets to relax, heal, and thrive — it's not waging war against itself. By eating foods that don't fit your system, you are literally expending unnecessary energy on yourself.

For those of us with autoimmune issues these two are HUGE for managing or eliminating our symptoms and relapses.

Eggs, Nuts, and Seeds

Excluding eggs, nuts, and seeds gives your digestive system a break and takes out potential sources of belly bacteria (SIBO) and stress caused by foods that are difficult to break down and dig the nutritional elements out of.

Caffeine and Alcohol

The Reset excludes caffeine and alcohol because they are unnecessary to a thriving system. They can literally fuel the inflammatory fire by adding acid to your system. By cutting these two out you will give your liver and adrenal glands a break from working so hard to constantly detox and balance your system. These two are really about the energy expended to filter them out.

Non-Gluten Grains

Non-gluten grains can be majorly tricky for a body. They can tripwire a gluten response and hinder healing. They are often consumed in amounts that are at a major imbalance in overall nutrition and are converting to glucose (sugar) in a system. They can work in small, balanced amounts but the key here is to allow time and space for healing and then see how your body truly responds to them.

Chocolate or Raw Cacao

These can be delightful and wonderful for a body when they are the real deal of 72% dark or higher, minus refined sugars. Although true dark cacao has wonderful antioxidants they run on the acidic side of the food spectrum so are best left out for a bit in order to quiet internal fires and allow healing.

Refined or Concentrated Sugars (honey, raw or otherwise, maple syrup, and molasses)

Sugars of any kind can be a landmine of metabolic issues and though real sugars do have some benefit, this is a category that needs to be kept in check regardless of real or refined.

Legumes (beans, peas, lentils, peanuts) Although these can be packed with wonderful nutrients they are also difficult to digest, retrieve the nutrients from or, for those of us with autoimmune issues, properly process metabolically.

Nightshades, Herbs and Spices that are Seed- or Nightshade-based

Seed-based spices: anise seed, annatto seed, black caraway, celery seed, coriander, cumin, dill seed, fennel seed, fenugreek, mustard seed, nutmeg, poppy seed, sesame seed;
Nightshade spices: capsicums, cayenne, chili pepper flakes, chili powder, curry, paprika, red pepper. Nightshades are a category of plants that includes tomatoes,

potatoes (not sweet potato), eggplant, goji berries, and any peppers (sweet or spicy). These are difficult to digest and can cause intestinal issues or tripwire autoimmune issues in a big way.

The first five days you will not be eating any of the "No" Foods, you'll just eat your Five Day Menu of batch-cooked foods.

You are never to go hungry on the Reset. You can eat any and all of the foods you have prepared — aside from smoothies and fruits these are reserved only to the morning time slot — if you are hungry, eat. If you're not hungry go minimal but don't skip meals.

One of the goals of the Reset is to navigate to a place of conversation with your body. What does it say it needs? If hungry, eat. If it's not, simply fuel it at meal times minimally, don't force feed yourself. Remember, it takes time for the physical body to catch up to everything we are doing to or for it. Some bodies will crave and need the nutrients introduced. Some have extreme hunger on the Reset because the body is receiving satiating nutrients for the first time in a long time or perhaps ever … for other bodies they aren't very hungry because the nutrients are satiating and they don't need as much. Whatever happens with your hunger levels, honor it and know it is correct for you.

My first Reset I ate three sweet potatoes a day plus the menu. My body was coming from a place of nutrient deficiency and malnourishment due to my thyroid issues, IBS, and Celiac. That tapered off over time. Just know that there is no single way to experience the Reset. There are typically two tracks that occur and neither are wrong, it's simply a matter of where your personal body is coming from and all the foods support healing and the progress to better.

On day six you begin to add back a serving of foods from your "no" list. You'll spend three days on each new add-in food. You'll simply layer the "no" foods into one of your meals, one at a time.

Keep a journal and take notes on everything you notice in your body after you add a "no" back in. If you have no reaction to your new introduction in the three days, you can move on to the next category of "no" foods.

Reactions look like many things. Again, there is no single absolute answer. Some of us will breakout with acne, or one pimple, others will have a bit of a heat rash, some will have bloating, others will be running for the bathroom. This is truly where the learning begins. You'll begin to cultivate awareness of and conversing with your personal system. Note-taking is imperative in this process. Anything off is off. The level or amount of that will drastically differ per person. Some people will have a reaction within 15 to 20 minutes, for others it will be on day three. This is where you begin to crack your personal food code. By the end of your 41 days you'll have a journal full of notes and be able to see patterns in your personal body that you can choose to abide by or not.

After years of Reset-style eating I know that some things will give me a mild reaction and from time to time I'm willing to "take the hit" as it's small and it will quietly make its way through my body. Other foods I avoid like the plague because of the amount of recovery time and issues they present in my body (hello, brown rice, corn and gluten). I have no desire to feel that awful or put my body through that pain and recovery.

Honor the Three Days of Re-Entry

Remember, your intestines are 23 feet long. It literally takes food you have consumed three to four days to fully pass all the way through your digestive tract. It takes time for things to work their way through and it may be on day three that something presents itself. After you introduce a new food take note of mood, energy levels, bloating, gas, discomfort, headaches, acne, rashes, and bowel movements from the moment you eat something new to the end of day three. A reaction in any of these areas can mean that the food is not a fit for you. The degree to which you experience any symptoms will let you know just how not-a-fit it is for you. Anytime I or my kids have something crop up I count back three to four days and see if there was anything new or out of the ordinary that was eaten. I usually find an affirmative answer there.

If you have symptoms, stop eating the new food and wait until symptoms subside before moving on to the next add-in. Yes, it could take longer than 41 days to truly identify what will work and what will not work for your system.

Side Note

How do I know if it's a reaction or not, or if it might even be a virus? You'll need to use your knowledge of yourself and your discernment, intellect, and gut instincts. If it's extreme, like vomiting or fever, it's viral or bacterial sickness/infection. Always tend to your body as you see fit and seek care if and when you need to. The Reset is simply whole real foods and will have some detox, cleansing elements to it but they are all typically minimal. If there is something major in your health, always seek care from a doctor.

The First Two Weeks

In the first two weeks of the Reset your body will be transitioning from toxin-laden to a clean machine. Your body will use any or all methods of ridding your system of these toxins (chemicals, metals, synthetic ingredients, glutens, and sugars). There is definitely a "die off" and cleansing period. This process all depends on where your system is coming from prior. You may be on multiple medications, supplements, OTC meds, fast food, soda, three or more caffeinated beverages a day, etc. You may already be eating clean and just want to know if all the real ingredients you eat are a fit for you or not. The more toxic your system is, the more intense the cleansing process can be.

The cleansing process takes place most intensely in the first five days of your Reset. Symptoms can include what may feel like sinus issues or catching a cold, diarrhea, constipation, acne, extreme fatigue, or headaches. Yes, you want to avoid these in the long run and will make a note of these reactions when you begin your add-ins on day six, but as bad stuff pushes through your system in your first five days, it can look like all the red flags. It's often referred to as an "acid drop." Be kind with the process and ride it out.

What you might experience

<u>**Days 1 - 3**</u>______Caffeine Headaches
__________**What you can do to help:**
Rest more when and where you can, go to bed earlier, take a nap, meditate. Up your hydration with water and lemon water, take an epsom salt bath to support the hydration and detox or use frankincense, lemon, peppermint, or lavender essential oils on your temples, forearms, and feet — a couple of drops of each, three times a day.

<u>**Days 1 - 4**</u>______Acid reflux or heartburn after drinking lemon water in the morning
__________**What you can do to help:**
Decrease the amount of lemon in the water from a half of a lemon to a quarter of a fresh lemon in your warm water in the morning. For two to four weeks then work your way back up to half a lemon.

<u>**Days 1 - 4**</u>______Upset stomach, bloating, or gas after drinking kombucha
__________**What you can do to help:**
Decrease the amount of kombucha you are drinking at a time to 2 oz. for two to four

weeks then work your way to to 4 oz. and then possibly 6 oz.

Days 3 - 4_________Cold or flu like symptoms. This is the period known as *die off* in your initial detox as the majority of foods, chemicals, and additives leave your system. They will choose whatever route to exit they can: sinuses, bowels, sweat glands, etc. You may have small headaches, sniffles, sneezes, mild diarrhea, fatigue. These are normal, appropriate, and healthy ways for a system to flush toxins out.
__________**What you can do to help:** Rest more when and where you can, go to bed earlier, take a nap, meditate. Up your hydration with water and lemon water, take as many epsom salt baths as you need to to support the hydration and detox or use oregano or ginger essential oils in a carrier oil on your feet, a couple of drops of each, three times a day. Day five things should be cleared up. If it's feverish or nauseous … that's the flu. If anything lasts past day 5 check in with your doctor(s).

Days 1 - 5______Fatigue

_________**What you can do to help:**
Rest more when and where you can, go to bed earlier, take a nap, meditate. Up your hydration with water and lemon water, take an epsom salt bath to support the hydration and detox or use peppermint, lime, and melaleuca (tea tree), vetiver or frankincense essential oils on your hands, forearms, and feet, a couple of drops of each, three times a day. If you are a www.unicornwellnessstudio.com member, you can also search your account for specific videos to assist energetic balance with the key words and phrases 'full stretch,' 'restorative,' 'rest,' or 'restoration.' Use these workouts one to five times in this time period.

Days 1 - 14_________Possible constipation

_________**What you can do to help:**
Focus on being fully hydrated with half of your bodyweight in ounces of water a day.

If you are currently at that level, drink a little more. You need ample hydration to process the amounts of fiber you are consuming on the Reset. Take epsom salt baths to support the hydration and detox or use peppermint, lime, and melaleuca (tea tree), vetiver or frankincense essential oils on your hands, forearms, and feet, a couple of drops of each, three times a day. If you are a matandkitchen.com member, you will want to use any detox-specific workouts you have to help assist the flushing process and intestinal massage. Search your account for specific videos with the key words and phrases 'detox,' 'digestion,' 'rotation,' or 'twist.' Use these workouts two to six times this week.

Days 21 - 27 Potential emotional meltdown — for some this week is a big one emotionally. Typically week four, **Days 28 - 34,** is the highest point of gluten detox but I have witnessed a significant percentage of participants have the emotional breakdown for the breakthrough happens in week three, **Days 21 - 27.**

What you can do to help: The basics of supportive self-care are always the starting point. Take epsom salt baths to support the hydration and detox, use lime and melaleuca (tea tree), vetiver or frankincense essential oils on your hands, forearms, and feet, a couple of drops of each, three times a day. If you are a www.unicornwellnessstudio.com member, you will want to use any detox specific workouts you have to help assist the flushing process and intestinal massage. Search your account for specific videos with the key words and phrases 'detox,' 'digestion,' 'rotation,' or 'twist.' Use these workouts two to six times this week.

Days 28 - 34   Emotional meltdown — this is the highest point of gluten detox for the body. It has not fully exited a system for another four to seven weeks but this is where you feel it the most. You may crave or have dreams about gluten and the bigger the emotional wave that comes this week, the bigger your body's issue with gluten. It's incredibly clear and useful information in the process. This is truly a potential moment for a breakdown to the breakthrough.

__________**What you can do to help:** The basics of supportive self-care are always the starting point. Take epsom salt baths to support the hydration and detox, use lime and melaleuca (tea tree), vetiver or frankincense essential oils on your hands, forearms, and feet, a couple of drops of each, three times a day. If you are a www.unicornwellnessstudio.com member, you will want to use any detox specific workouts you have to help assist the flushing process and intestinal massage. Search your account for specific videos with the key words and phrases 'detox,' 'digestion,' 'rotation,' or 'twist.' Use these workouts two to six times this week.

Hydration

It's imperative to be fully hydrated on the Reset. Your body will be doing a full clean sweep of things it has stashed for years and needs water to truly assist the process. Be diligent with hydrating your body with half of your body weight in ounces of water a day. Some bodies may even need more. A small percentage of those who embark on the Reset experience constipation in the first two weeks of the Reset if your body has been at a deficit of fiber or isn't being supported with enough hydration to pass and process the fiber it will begin to take in on the Reset. Try not to be discouraged. Begin to practice radical self-care, hang in there, hydrate, rest, take epsom baths, and if needed: communicate in the private groups on Facebook. If it persists past Day 16 there are things we can adjust and try. Typically, it simply passes. Pun intended.

Healing Takes Time

Getting better can be messy. Budget time for some additional rest during the first portion of the Reset. Focus on hydration — half of your bodyweight in ounces of water a day — to flush your system out. Take a bath in Epsom salts when you're not feeling well — they aid in the detox process.

Add 1-2 cups of Epsom salts to a warm bath. A 15-minute soak helps detox and a full 40 minutes hydrates you as well.

Most people go through the Reset with very few of these reactions. However, it's all in the spectrum of *normal* in the transition to a clean system. Use common sense, if you drink a ton of caffeine prior to the Reset, do not try to cold turkey it. Pare down your consumption and start the Reset when your system is ready to do without.

As you go through the process it can be helpful to know what's still in your system, and what's leaving that may make you feel less than fabulous.

Dairy, chocolate, legumes, nightshades, eggs, and nuts exit the system in three to four days.

Sugars exit in 21 to 26 days. This includes alcohol and all non-gluten grains.

Coffee takes 26 days to exit but its effects on the adrenal glands can last much longer.

Gluten takes a full eight to 11 weeks to leave your system.

Exit Time Line	
Days 3 - 4	Dairy, Chocolate, Legumes, Nightshades, Eggs and Nuts
Days 21 - 26	Alcohol and Non-Gluten Grains
Day 26	Coffee
Days 56 - 77	Gluten Grains – Barley, Wheat and Rye

Post Reset

You'll choose whether you leave your "no" foods out of your life for good or if they're worth the discomfort in moderation. It's all about education and choices. Cracking your food code is empowering and takes the mystery out of *why* your body functions as it does or is the way it is. By knowing what triggers unwell responses in your body you have the power and the choice to continue those things or release them. You have the power of choice when it comes to your body and its health. You'll have the tools when it comes to food at the end of your Reset to navigate yourself towards your best health!

How to Re-Introduce the 'No' Foods

Add foods back in this order:

Day 6 - Eggs — Only add one egg at a time. If you want to go the optimal route try just the yolk on Day 6, only the egg white on Day 7, and the entire egg Day 8. The whites of the egg are where the bacteria are; the yolks house vitamins D, A, E, and K along with the omega-3s (yay for good fats!), the antioxidants lutein and zeaxanthin. It's true that the whites have fabulous B12 but the pesky bacteria might not work for your body.

If eggs have been an issue for your system in the past, here are some tips to try.

- Make sure your eggs are organic and pasture raised. Cage free is *not* the same as pasture raised and the cleanliness and respect to how they are raised does matter. If you can get them from a friend or local farm, do so.
- Try duck eggs - Yes, they will take a bit more effort to find but they are notoriously easier to digest and an excellent match for sensitive systems. They are also divine to cook and bake with down the road. They are much larger than a traditional chicken egg and their good fat content reflects that with more protein and more omega- 3s. They are delicious.
- Try small eggs - Quail eggs have become much easier to find and in addition to their adorably small size they pack a protein punch. Quail

eggs have more protein than a
chicken egg as well as more B1.
They also can help fight allergy
symptoms due to the ovomucoid
protein found in them. Their small
size cuts down on the overall work
your digestive system has to do with
them as well as cutting down on the
amount of bacteria in them.

Day 9 - Caffeine — Drink an espresso, or
a cup of green or black tea. You can do the
same one on all three days or try
something different each day.

As with everything we ingest, the type
matters and different things will work for
different bodies. Coffee has been
demonized for generations when it comes
to *best* healing practices, but the fact is, it
has some wonderful health benefits. Green
tea can be unbelievably magical for some,
for those of us with sensitive systems we
need to avoid it and though tea caffeine is
more gentle on a nervous system, some of
us react more intensely to it than coffee.

I teach the details of tea vs. coffee in my 30 Days to be a Moon Momma online course but here are some basics:

- One shot of espresso has an average of 70 mg of caffeine as compared to 370 mg in a cup of drip coffee … needless to say I only drink espresso.
- Drip coffee is far more acidic than espresso. Acidic = bad, akalline = good, when it comes to food and drink. The Reset aims for a balance with a skew towards alkaline. A little acid is fine, too much creates an environment for sickness to make a home in your body.
- If you choose to try drip coffee aim for organic. If it's not organic it's often roasted in flavors and flavoring that are anything but good for you. Non organic coffees can also be cross contaminated with gluten as well. Green coffee beans are an excellent choice overall for the healthiest bean.
- Green tea should be avoided by those with anemia, anxiety issues, liver disease, or those who are pregnant or diabetic. It can cause

stomach problems, racing heartbeat, diarrhea, and headaches. It has about 35 mg of caffeine per cup.

- Tea in general is more kind to our nervous system. The leaves are aged. Whereas coffee beans are "young" caffeine, tea is an "older" caffeine. Black tea contains approximately 47 mg of caffeine per cup, but on a personal note if I drink black tea I'm up all night, but a double shot of espresso … I'm fine (all before 2:30 p.m. of course).
- Always aim for organic in your tea and coffee. Especially tea. Most tea leaves are not washed prior to aging and packaging. Conventional tea is a landmine of pesticides and chemicals. Organic tea leaves are not only chemical free but also guaranteed to be washed prior to aging.
- Always read the label, especially your tea, during the Reset. Tea is a super sneaky place where chemicals, fillers, and gluten can hide. These are often listed as natural flavors or

natural flavoring. This is a labeling issue — sometimes these things can genuinely be lemon zest or herbs but often they are code for thickeners and preservatives that wreak havoc on your system. During the Reset please drink only organic tea or coffee with listed known ingredients. Avoid natural flavoring or natural flavors.

- Bonus note — Avoid decaf coffee at all costs unless you have access to one that has gone through a water process (which is rare). In general decaf coffee has been put through a highly chemical process to take the caffeine out of the bean that is far more deleterious to your system than the actual caffeine. Again, there is research as to the benefits of coffee caffeine for a body. It's always a matter of what is a fit for your personal system. For example, I can drink espresso, not drip coffee, or black or green tea. The only way to know what works for you is to test it out … however, heavy chemicals don't ever work for anyone in the long run. Avoid the biggies, like decaf coffee.

Day 12 - Nuts — You can have any raw, unroasted, unsalted nut, but no more than seven at a time. You are welcome to test a nut-butter, just keep it raw, make sure there's nothing else in it aside from the nut, unroasted, unsalted, and no sugars or oils. As always, make sure they are organic. The chemicals on non-organic nuts can do more damage than the nut itself.

If you know you have a highly sensitive system, sprout the raw nuts first or go with the nut butter, as the processing of it can be easier on your digestive system.

To sprout nuts simply soak them in a bowl of water overnight. This allows easier digestion and easier access and absorption of their nutrients. You can try three different kinds on the three days. Different nuts may produce different results. I suggest Brazil nuts, cashews and walnuts. And yes, I know a cashew is not an actual nut, it's a drupe, it always ends up in this category anyhow and because it's a drupe (closer to a fruit in many respects) it's easier to digest and tolerate.

Please no peanuts at this point. Peanuts are not actually nuts, they are legumes and from a digestive perspective we are testing these Day 36-38. Wait until then for the sake of healing and clear answers on whether or not they work for your system.

Day 15 - Seeds — Add a teaspoon of hemp, chia, flax, pumpkin, sesame, or sunflower seeds to one meal or snack in your day. Keep them raw, organic, salt- and roasting-free. You are welcome to try sunbutter if you have one that is only the blended sunflower seeds. No added sugars or additional ingredients. The digestive issue with seeds is that they are so small, if there is gut damage of any kind, they get caught in the fissure, holes, and tears. They're also difficult for your system to dig the nutrients out of.

Soaking or sprouting nuts and seeds assist in making the nutrients more available to your gut while decreasing the amount of work your body has to do to in order to digest them. Soaking and sprouting simply means to let them soak in water six to eight hours prior to cooking or eating.

Chia seeds and hemp seeds are my picks for this category. These two are the only plant-based proteins with complete amino acids.

***BONUS RECIPE** This is a great place to explore homemade hemp milk, listed in the Reset recipes, or unfiltered, organic flax oil. This is a case where the processing aids in the potential to access nutrients and ease digestive distress and actually increase nutrient absorption.

Day 18 - Raw Cacao — Add a teaspoon in your smoothie or eat it by itself. Raw cacao is the raw, pure form of chocolate. It is a wonderful antioxidant and will allow you to know if chocolate works minus the sugar. This is what women crave during PMS, we crave the magnesium that acts as a muscle relaxant in cacao — not the processed-refined-sugar-laden milk chocolate we've been downing for generations.

Although you'll only be testing one tablespoon at a time in the next three days if it works for you in the testing phase, you can add an additional teaspoon in the days to come for optimal benefit. The benefits of consuming *2 tablespoons of raw cacao 3x a week are:*

- 20 times more antioxidants than a 1/2 cup of blueberries
- An actual mood boost because it contains anandamide — often called the bliss molecule because it creates a feeling of euphoria in the body, No, it's not pretend … we are happier when we eat cacao.
- A serotonin boost - Serotonin is the "happiness maker" when it comes to our bodies. It balances moods, social behavior, sex drive, and sexual function, appetite, digestion, and

sleep. We hear so much about regulating it in our brain, but 80-90% of our serotonin transmitters are located in our gut. In our actual belly and digestive system — hence the importance of a healthy, leak free, balanced gut … the *entire* point of the Reset! Feminine systems tank out on serotonin during PMS, making raw cacao a super choice when it comes to PMS solutions and the overall balancing of hormones for fitness and wellness results.

- Flavonol - Flavonol provides antioxidant effects that protect your heart from heart disease, increase circulation, and reduce the risk of stroke.
- Sneaky Sunscreen - Here's a cool kicker for health, raw cacao actually protects your skin from UV rays *from the inside out!* It's internal sunscreen when consumed consistently.
- Fiber - Raw cacao is packed with fiber so it's excellent for your digestive system and bowel movements. Make sure to keep up

on hydration -— half of your bodyweight in ounces of water a day — to keep your system happy with the upswing in fiber if you do add cacao consistently to your life.

Many ancient tribal communities considered raw cacao as deep healing, feminine medicine. It was actually called the drink of the gods.

And yes, there is a difference between cacao and cocoa. Cacao is the raw form of chocolate cold pressed and unroasted to retain all the nourishing elements. Cocoa is raw cacao that has been roasted at high temperatures that destroy its nutritional value. Cocoa is also often treated or combined with alkali, which adjusts the color and consistency of the cacao but also destroys the health benefits of it.

*** After day 26 feel free to try my bonus recipe for hot cacao! It's dreamy and powerful if all the elements work for your system! It's wonderful prior to bedtime as well because of the relaxing magnesium.

Day 21 - Alcohol — Celebrate today and add in one to four ounces of organic red, white, rosé, or plum wine or try a Silver/Blanco tequila or Mezcal.

Avoid anything from a gluten grain (beer, most gin, or most vodka). Potato vodka is to be avoided as it is a nightshade and corn vodka or sake (rice) would technically be a non-gluten grain and we're not there yet.

Any alcohol that is clear, by Traditional Chinese Medicine, is best for the body and can be tested post Reset. Day 21-23 stick to my recommendations and raise a glass to your health!

BONUS NOTE In week three — THIS WEEK — You may open up your menu to any clean, pasture-raised, wild-caught, 100% grass-fed animal proteins. Be very careful with the 100% grass-fed proteins. Proteins will be labeled grass-fed but are not 100% grass-fed unless labeled as such. This means, it's a waste of money and not completely *clean*.

Proteins labeled *grass-fed* but not *100% grass-fed* are grass-fed up until 120 days prior to slaughter. This is called *finishing* or finish *feeding*. To fatten them up. In my opinion this is a complete waste of the prior grass-feeding for the animal and to our nutrient benefit. In addition, if you have a sensitive system and react to grain-fed animals (as I do) your system won't register them as clean either. They are a waste of money. It's nothing but a feel-good-marketing-ploy label to be avoided for the sake of your pocketbook and wellness.

Stick with the simple preparations: only coconut or olive oil plus the herbs already listed here in your Reset menu. This will make eating out or packing meals easier. There are many wild-caught canned sardines and anchovies out there to make life more diverse and simple.

Keep red meats minimal. Your system may very much need the iron, fats, and protein from it, but there's no need to go overboard.

***You do not need to wait three to four days as an *add-in* if you choose to add additional proteins.

Day 24 - Sugars — In these three days you get to try one teaspoon of raw honey, pure maple syrup, or molasses. Add it to your coffee or tea if you got to keep them or to your morning smoothie — or just eat it off the spoon. These particular sweets can be beneficial to your body so we test these during the Reset and you can keep anything that works.

Raw honey offers incredible antibacterial and antimicrobial benefits. Maple syrup provides an incredible amount of manganese and magnesium, and molasses is packed with B6, iron, selenium and calcium.

You can test refined sugars after the Reset if you like, but at this stage your system is essentially free of the sugars that do damage and provide zero nutrient value, so why go adding them back in?

Once refined sugar has fully exited your system, sugar cravings can stop. Sugar definitely has a *feed the demon* element. For many of us, we need to break up and stay away from refined sugars because once you're back on the sugar wagon of doping your system for that rush … you're forever chasing that dragon. Sugar cravings call to be fed with more and more and more sugar. Sugar truly is a drug, so once it's out, honor your body and keep it out. There is no nutritional or emotional value to it at all.

Sugar cravings can and do stop once you rid your body of it. You can still have sweets and treats, without the monster of refined sugars rearing its nasty head. There's a beautiful world of raw honey, maple syrup and coconut sugar out there to play with and enjoy that don't wreak havoc on your insulin levels.

Don't make the mistake of using agave. It's nothing but a beautiful marketing job well done that makes us think it's a *healthy* sugar option. It's worse than refined white sugar. It's highly processed and heat treated and is just as bad as High Fructose Corn Syrup. Agave syrup, in its original form may not initially raise insulin levels and scores low on the Glycemic Index, but it's all about the long term effect of it in our body and on our system.

Agave sweetener is 85% fructose which causes major damage in the long run to your metabolic system by causing insulin resistance, raising the risk of Type 2 Diabetes, belly fat accumulation, and higher LDLs (the bad cholesterol). In a nutshell, stay far away from it. It's a complete marketing scam.

**BONUS NOTE - the body cannot distinguish where a sugar (fructose or glucose) comes from. This is why fruits are limited on the Reset. Sweet is sweet and though better is better and sweet coming from raw honey or a piece of fruit is exponentially better than using agave or eating a candy bar, our bodies are not built to run on sugars. We are built to function and thrive on veggies and clean proteins. Sweets, in any form should be minimal and in addition to our meals, not the bulk of them. When we overdo sugars, in any form, we throw off the optimal internal balance of our body.

Day 27 - Dairy — In these three days you get to add one to three ounces of dairy. This is another add-in to navigate thoughtfully. Our human systems are not actually built to digest cow's milk. It is truly the masterful work of the dairy council that has convinced generations that we need it for strong bones and ample calcium. It's simply not accurate. But, bravo to that marketing campaign and lobbyist dollars.

The casein (protein) in cow dairy may be plentiful, but our digestive tracts are not calibrated to it. Dairy, in an overabundance, generates mucus, inflammation, and muckiness in our systems. I do believe in moderation and that most sources of food can help your personal system to balance, hence, cracking your own food code. Keep this in the forefront of your mind as you add in dairy. It can be a tricky food, similar to sugar, that if you go full steam on this train you enter into an addictive cycle of it, which is real.

Try goat and sheep milk products first. These typically cause fewer intestinal problems than cow's milk products. The chemical makeup is different and free of casein.

Cheeses, kefir, and yogurt may have a different response than milk. You'll need to play with these. I suggest adding in goat or sheep yogurt, cheese, then milk, then move to a beautiful crafted cheese. Always #goreal when it comes to your food. Quality matters.

Always choose organic, hormone-free, hand-crafted varieties of dairy when possible and read the labels to make sure there are no additives, sugars or

unpronounceable or unknown ingredients
in your dairy choices.

IMPORTANT NOTE
You are heading into week four of the
Reset. If gluten is an issue for your body,
you're going to get some major signals this
week.

Week four is the highest point of detox for
gluten grains. It takes eight to 11 weeks for
gluten to fully exit a system and although
you are not completely free and clear of
gluten, at this point, if it's a no-no for your
system you may very well experience a
massive emotional meltdown this week
(and sometimes prior in week 3, because
bodies are incredibly unique). Honor what's
coming up.

Take extra care of yourself this week with
self-care, additional sleep, rest, meditation,
epsom salt baths, and hydration. Keep
your journal close by and write it out when
things get emotional. It's a huge sign of
healing. Honor it and try to embrace it.

You may have a lot of anger, frustration or sadness surface. You may feel mood swings, anxiety, or depression or, yay, both. Your skin may break out and most often, you may dream of all things gluten or have real cravings for barley, wheat and rye products you can think of.

I've coached myself, my kids, my husband, friends, and enough clients through this to know it's real. Honor it. I always look at it as a wonderful blessing. When the breakdown is so loud and clear the breakthrough and healing are just around the corner. For more information on things you might experience while on the Reset, reference the section on *What You Might Experience* just a few pages back .

Day 30 - Non-Gluten Grains — Try a ½ cup serving of white rice, buckwheat, or amaranth added to any meal or snack. If you are currently healing autoimmune issues a ½ cup may be far too much, try a tablespoon.

The reaction that always comes with this group of add-ins is the shock and awe of white rice.

This is another one of those where we've been fed a line of baloney for generations, through marketing, that it's awful for us. One of the things I really want readers to learn from the Reset is that real is always a good choice when it comes to food, that everyone of us thrives slightly differently and that by cracking our personal food code we honor our personal needs for our best health. Don't buy into the mass media false paradigms that we've been sold for generations. Figure out what works for you, now, and honor that. Hold tight to your personal wellness revolution and march to the beat of your own, whole, clean food drum.

There's nothing wrong with carbs, simple or complex. They are both necessary to our overall wellness.

White rice is actually a cleaner food source than brown rice … because of the processing it goes through. The nutshell of this conversation is brown rice contains phytic acid as well as trace amounts of arsenic. Both make it difficult to digest, dirty, and harmful to the gut and are both removed in the milling process that turns it into white rice. White rice is a lovely resource of constructive carbs and cools the temperment of the body in terms of Traditional Chinese Medicine.

White rice is my personal choice when it comes to grains. It resides in the *do no harm* category.

Corn also falls into the non-gluten grain category. Watch for inflammation as a "no" sign for you. Most often in the manifestation of arthritis, achy and swollen joints. Keep an eye on how your toes, fingers, and knees feel after this one. Homemade organic popcorn is easiest to test for this one throw some coconut oil and pink salt on it and you're in business!

Also be aware that even non-gluten grains can tripwire a gluten reaction in the body. Some systems, in particular those with autoimmune issues, are so damaged and *mad* at gluten that they mistake even non-gluten grains and fire an autoimmune response. This is a completely per person issue. Some will have it (I do), others will not. Again, another serious vote for abiding by your food code for your best health. Yes, it is possible to heal past this in time and reintroduce non-gluten grains down the road. Each person is beautifully different in this aspect as well.

Test your add ins, see how your body responds. Take notes, honor it and potentially retest three to 24 months down the road.

Day 33 - Gluten Grains — If you already know that gluten does not work for you, d*o not test it!* For those of you that are already feeling better without them, going gluten-free or avidly working to heal Celiac — now is the time to check in with yourself, your gut, your intuition, and make the decision to test it or not. *If you do not choose to test gluten grains* you're more than halfway to its full exit point. It takes eight to 11 weeks for gluten grains to fully exit the body. Gluten detox is real and it's a long haul. You're currently past the hardest point of it's exit (week #4).

If you do choose to add it in in these three days a little dab will do ya. Go easy with it, try a half a piece of wheat, rye, or barley toast.

Remember to watch out for the more subtle symptoms with gluten. Yes, the gastrointestinal signs are the easiest to register: bloating, gas, diarrhea, abdominal pain, cramping, stabbing or squeezing sensations, or constipation in the following days. But few people know that gluten sensitivity is one of the leading contributors to depression and anxiety. It also often causes *brain fog*: difficulty focusing or remembering things along with extreme fatigue.

Gluten is very particular per person, so honor your body and take ample notes in your journal if you test it. It's sneaky. I cannot tell you how many times clients say

"I didn't have any digestional issue with gluten" … meanwhile they don't always see or register the downturn of other areas of their wellness, in particular depression, anxiety, bloating/weight gain and sleep disruptions.

I don't have anything against gluten, aside from the fact that it's been modified and hybridized for generations. It's no longer a *real* food. There is a real problem in how it's been produced for generations in the United States and we are just now dealing with health related issues of it.

Our systems were never built or meant to have the bulk of our nutrients come from grains. At best, if we can tolerate them and find we thrive with them, it's supplemental to veggies and a clean bit of protein. Culturally we are dealing with two main issues with gluten, the quality of it and the quantity at which our culture consumes it. It's nearly impossible to get *clean* gluten in the United States, hence why many gluten sensitive or intolerant or even Celiacs can ingest gluten when in other countries. Our sources are so laden in chemicals it's no longer real.

Then we have the quantity of grains that we, as a culture, consume — which are unbelievably disproportionate to how a body thrives.

Give gluten some thought. Test it if you need to or skip it if you'd like to make it to the full exit at 11 weeks and see how your personal system feels. The Reset is a food adventure and education with the end goal being you feeling amazing and thriving and empowering yourself to make choices to work with your body rather than against it.

Also know that being gluten free isn't about swapping gluten for overly processed gluten-free products. Being gluten-free doesn't inherently or instantly make you healthy. Anchoring in whole real foods and abiding by your personal food code makes you healthy and vibrant. Wellness isn't about a label. It's about clean and real.

Day 36 - Legumes — Legumes can be a good source of plant-based protein, but, sadly, are also very difficult to digest and contribute to generating and feeding bad bacteria, through their lectin known as agglutinin and phytates, in your gut. Through the Reset, we work very hard to establish a balance of good and bad bacteria. The last thing we need is anything that feeds the bad bacteria in our gut.

Legumes directly contribute to *leaky gut* — the creation of damage, tears, and holes in your digestive tissues/walls that allow for toxin build up and sometimes the passage of toxins directly into the bloodstream because of the holes and tears — because of legumes high concentration of slow burning carbs, something that is often marked as their major benefit.

The nutrients in legumes can be made easier to access and digest by soaking or sprouting them prior to cooking. Soaking or sprouting simply means letting them sit in water six to eight hours prior to cooking.

This is an excellent route to take when testing them.

Although plant-based proteins are touted as an excellent nutrient source they are not (aside from chia and hemp) complete proteins with all essential amino acids. This is part of what makes being vegan or vegetarian a bit more complicated. Most people are not educated or aware enough to combine foods properly and are simply creating hormone and nutrient imbalance in their bodies in the long run because of missing elements in their food sources. If post Reset you do find your body can thrive with a fully vegetarian or vegan diet you will need to take additional care and education that you are completing the amino acids for your body to thrive long term.

For this add-in try a half cup of snow peas or green beans. These are the easiest to digest, with the best nutrient profiles. If you'd like to test a third, black beans, lentils, or a small handful of raw organic peanuts or peanut butter are fair game.

Keep them organic, salt- and roasting-free and consider sprouting them prior.

Legumes with edible pods; green beans, snow peas, snap peas, Chinese long beans (also known as asparagus beans) and hyacinth beans, have a different nutrient profile than other legumes and are often better tolerated by sensitive and autoimmune systems, plus, have more nutrients than other legumes. These are my recommendations for legume add-ins.

Day 39 - Nightshades — This food category is left till the very end because they can have the sneakiest, most subtle, and oddest reactions. These are typically only an issue to those with autoimmune issues, leaky gut, or other leaky gut-related diseases. Nightshades are vegetables that are a part of the Solanaceae plant family. They include potatoes, tomatoes, eggplants, goji berries, and peppers and include a long list of herbs and spices, the most common being paprika and cayenne pepper.

The science as to why these can trigger issues is a bit more complicated than other add-in foods. The short answer is the presence of alkaloids found in them that can be stashed in the body than released in times of stress that just make a bad health situation worse.

Typical reactions can look like a spectrum of things like heartburn, joint pain, IBS symptoms, gastrointestinal distress and circulation issues, or in my case, a feeling like you hungover the next day. My biggest autoimmune issue is fatigue. It took me a long time to pin down this reaction. When I'm healthy and bolstered I can manage tomatoes and bell peppers, but if I've been triggered with other foods, I ditch these instantly.

Nightshades can simply tripwire autoimmune flare-ups, big time.

When testing this add-in try a half cup of tomatoes, bell peppers, potatoes (remember sweet potatoes are not nightshades), or eggplant, cooked or raw.

One teaspoon of goji berries or 1/4
teaspoon of any of the nightshade-based
herb. I recommend going with the most
common ones first that you are likely to
encounter most often like paprika or
cayenne pepper.

Your Personal Food Adventure

I always encourage those embarking on
the Reset to set their mind to a different
spectrum and embrace it as a food
adventure. It's important to approach this
experience with a sense of open
heartedness and *not knowing*. It's
imperative during these 41 days to be a
student of your food and body and be
willing to be wrong and to learn, rather than
anticipate, pre-empt or *already know* how
things will shake out with your personal
food code.

The reality is, if you already knew your food
code, knew what fuel truly allowed you to

feel amazing *you wouldn't be considering
the Reset.*

Something has led you here. Something is
either quietly nagging you or loudly yelling
at you and you believe it to be sourced or
solved with food. Listen to your instincts.
Heed the call of your intuition and intellect.
You know yourself best and there is truth in
those messages.

Embrace this food adventure as a personal
science experiment. Keep the variables
minimal and controlled. Commit for 41
days, be diligent, plan and prepare, pack
meals and snacks so you're never caught
in a situation that will push you to
compromise the experiment. Forty-one
days is a blip in our glorious lives. Embrace
it as the time to experience something you
never have before and give it the
opportunity to usher you into an
unbelievably better life experience.

You body is capable and built to feel
amazing. You simply need to peel off the

layers of what does not work for your unique system.

You may find that some kinds of nuts or seeds are okay or that certain caffeine is tolerable while another is not (i.e. green tea and not coffee). You may find that white rice is the only grain that works for you. You may also find that the amount or frequency of foods affects you differently. This initial commitment to the unfolding of your best self offers a huge opportunity and an incredible baseline for your thrival.

The Reset gives you a strong base of knowledge to work with. You'll develop an incredible dialogue with your body that will guide you for a lifetime to keep you focused on your healthiest journey with food that no longer involves the latest news report, study, fad or *diet* — oh, how I cringe at that word.

Post Reset you will have something far more powerful than all of those things combined.

You will have you. You have your body. You have your experience. You have your personal dialogue with nutrients and fuel. In order to know what works for you all you need to do is try it — and observe what your body tells you about it.

Our bodies are meant to thrive.

They are brilliantly and beautifully designed to work,consistently, with minimal glitches. They are designed to send us warning signals. When we ignore those signals or simply don't know how to translate the signals we get, that's when our wellness declines in sneaky and subtle, or in some cases not-so-subtle, ways.

We are each empowered through the Reset to embrace abundant upswings and true wellness. We reclaim an education of ourselves that no one can take away from us.
We no longer allow external noise to influence our personal food code.
We allow space and time for healing and positive change through the Reset.

If you'd like support during your Reset journey join the private Facebook group, The Reset.

Check-in as often you need or want to. Set yourself up for success by choosing a time to do the Reset that's not a super stressful one — no big moves, projects, or job transitions. Keeping in mind there is no absolute perfect time, there will always be a holiday, a party, a birthday, a work meeting, a conference, etc. Embrace the idea that any time to start healing is a good time. Get all of your supplies in the house and batch cook in one big swoop prior to starting.

In a perfect world all of your Reset foods would be organic, chemical-free, hormone-free, and 100% grass-fed or pasture raised. However #betterisbetter If you don't have access or budget to support this, do as much organic and clean as you can.

Don't create yet another barrier to your best health with a perfection roadblock.

Do not make substitutions or additions to
the Reset menu.

This is very important.

If you know you are allergic or already
have issues with certain foods, i.e.
cauliflower, broccoli, cruciferous
vegetables, etc. leave them out. If it's
simply a matter of *like* or *dislike* I ask you to
truly approach the Reset as medicine and
suspend juvenile blocks such as likes or
dislikes. The Reset is an education in
nourishment and earth medicine vs.
emotional, comfort or entertainment eating.
It's for your greatest good in the long run,
it's not for your current comfort or
limitations.

Remember, magic happens outside of your
comfort zone and the moment you shout at
the universe you'll *never* do x, y or z …
that's the moment the universe decides to
offer you an education on always and
never.

Your taste buds will change and literally *reset* during this experience. Things you find you nearly could not stomach in the beginning — like the green smoothie or beets — you will crave by the end.

The Reset demonstrates the power of additives and our addictions to refined sugars. I ask you to keep an open mind. Twelve years of research, time, and thought went into developing the Reset. I choose foods that bolster, nourish, and heal your system in the shortest amount of time. Your Reset menu is all about bang-for-the-buck in the shortest amount of time with a perspective that combines an alkaline diet, Traditional Chinese Medicine and a Paleo perspective for healing and thrival.

I have no desire to see a particular food trend be born or pull from one diet "team" to another. I have every desire to see as many people as possible heal and thrive, love themselves and their bodies, feel amazing and make a positive impact on the world.

All constructive changes and powerful personal transitions happen outside of your comfort zone.

You've typically been eating what you like, what was near, most efficient, what you wanted, what sounded fun or entertaining, what was cheapest, or what someone else deemed *best* up to this point. These practices have cultivated your current health and fitness.

In order for your body to change, the food you eat must change.

Be willing to be wrong in order to become your best and healthiest self.

Batch Cooking

Batch cooking just means that you prep, chop, and pre-cook your ingredients or meals at one or two times in the week. You prepare multiple servings ahead of time.

You'll need to batch cook your Reset meals one day prior to starting the Reset, for the entire week. You'll prep everything and stash in containers to keep in your fridge so the day-to-day execution of your menu is simply a matter of grab and go or assembly — wherever and whenever you go!

You should never go hungry on the Reset or be caught by surprise. You'll need to take meals with you — eating out, depending on where you live, could be quite a challenge. Always be prepared in these 41 days for ultimate success in cracking your food code.

Batch cooking has long been a tactic of successful personal trainers and athletes. It is also how my family thrives on our busy schedules. I promise you, no one is busier than my household of four, all of which have food issues that need to be managed for our direct wellness. My husband and youngest are gluten sensitive, my oldest son has severe psoriasis that is only managed by diligently being gluten-, almond- and peanut-free and I have Celiac, IBS, and a thyroidectomy — food is literally my thrival and survival. If we can find time to prep, so can you.

Doing hard things is always about understanding their worth and making a commitment to it. You can always find a way, this I promise you. The universe will swoop into support your efforts and self-respect and self-care.

My family batch cooks every week. I make larger portions of each of our dinners so that everyone has leftovers for lunch the next day and on either Sunday or Monday I cut and prep all the raw veggies so we can either grab and assemble or cook. Batch cooking is actually more efficient in the long run. Instead of prepping and cooking for every meal, it's done at one time, than meals are simply a matter of assembly.

Batch cooking cuts down on the scramble and stress of eating. You know what you have, you don't want it to go to waste, you know you're doing something beautiful, protective, and proactive for the wellness of your body and there is a huge sense of accomplishment from preparing everything.

You will reap a sense of pride from your preparation!

Implementing this technique will change your health and therefore your life.

The first time you batch cook it could take up to four hours. It will be faster each time you do it! It takes practice and repetition to cultivate mastery — another reason the Reset menu is repetitive in this 41 days — and the speed at which you complete your batch cooking the first go round will have a lot to do with how kitchen- and cooking-savvy you are prior to this adventure.

I'll tell you straight up I rarely to never cooked prior to writing the Reset. It's something that my husband and I often laugh about now … I used to burn everything. I was terrified of cooking. I had an innate fear of food because I knew it tripwired all the awful things in my body. I avoided it at all costs because it was never rewarding….. and therefore I wasn't skilled at it.

I'm sharing this because many people are daunted by the concept of batch cooking — or any cooking at all — and I'm here to encourage you to make mistakes and to learn, because if I can do it, so can you.

When you finally begin to rock 'n roll with your batch cooking it should hover in the range of two hours.

The Menu

The menu below is designed specifically for the Reset. You get to eat as much of the food that you have prepped as you like. If you're starving … EAT! If you find yourself not hungry, go mellow. Eat your menu but it doesn't have to be large portions.

I don't count calories and neither should you

It creates stress in your system, both hormonal and digestive. If you are eating whole, real food there is truly no need to count, measure or weigh.

Listen and respond to your body. Eat when hungry. Stop when you are full.

For some of us, we are starving on the Reset. It may be the first time our bodies have been capable and able to get the nutrients we so badly need. Remember — my personal first Reset, I ate three entire sweet potatoes a day in addition to my meals. My body was screaming at me for more, more, more! I honored that and I fed it.

For others, the Reset food satiates a body's hunger for nutrients at such a bolstered level that it doesn't need much at all. Their bodies say a little is enough and isn't starving. For many people this is the case. Their systems are so used to gorging on empty nutrients — processed grains and sugars — that when they are finally fueled with nutrient-dense food it is shocked to be full.

Either way, the response of hunger or not, is normal.

The Reset grocery list included at the end of the recipes section is written for one and a half person.

Yup. I said a half person. I see the face you're making … I say one and a half person because some people are starving on the Reset and will need the extra food stashed in the fridge. Some people won't be hungry at all and won't need the extra. If this is the case, simply freeze the extra for the following week or share with someone!

It's also a *thing* that the Reset food will look so delicious and inviting to those you are with, partners, spouses, children, that they will want to partake of the food. This grocery list allows that to happen in a fluid way so you're not missing elements for your personal Reset.

Anyone can eat all the food on the Reset without actually *doing* the Reset. The Reset is a completely do-no-harm process. It's all whole, real, clean foods to bolster, nourish, heal, and template health in any body. I often refer to it as farm food because, in truth, that's what it is. Food straight from the earth as un-messed with as possible straight to your body.

The Social Aspect

As I mentioned prior, there is no perfect time to do the Reset. Neither you, nor I, live in a bubble. There will always be a holiday party, birthday, vacation, conference, or travel to deal with and navigate through.

Prepare for these endeavors by packing and taking your meals or snacks or eating prior or directly after. Focus on these celebrations and the event rather than the food that's there. Our food culture is an entirely other book. Take care of you, boo, on this wellness journey.

If you must go out to eat during your Reset; research restaurants and menus ahead of time. Try to choose where you are going rather than having to navigate a place someone else chose. If you have a catered event to attend, either pack your own things or call and ask questions. Ask for special things. Yup. You deserve it. Navigate the best you can in the particular environment that you are in. #betterisbetter but remember that you are doing the Reset to crack your food code and get answers for your well being. It's important. You're investing time and money into this experience, don't let something *other* derail it.

If you don't feel comfortable advocating for yourself with questions, research, or packed meals … there is a lesson here in and of itself. If people are rude or resistant to helping you discover your best food code, that's their problem, not a reflection of you. If you do go to restaurants, tell them you have food allergies rather than "I'm trying this thing." or the worst "I'm on a diet" (No, you're not).

Honor this exploration of your wellness, give it space, protect it. People in the U.S. hear allergy and understand the gravity of it. They will help you when they hear this, whereas if you make mention of a *diet* or *thing*…they will mock you as they enter the kitchen to place your order. Remember, going out to eat is a service industry, they are there to assist and serve you.

If you're lucky enough to be in Europe countries you'll experience something entirely different, with extensively labeled menus that make life incredibly easy to navigate. I can't speak to other countries just yet, you'll have to let me know!

There will also always be well-meaning family, friends, and colleagues who have an opinion about what you are doing for your wellness, and in particular with your food. Food is highly emotionally charged and often more so for others than for those willing to do the Reset.

My advice to you in this process is to **not** try and explain what it is you are doing and for goodness sakes **do not** try to convince anyone to do it with you.

Keep it simple. Do this for you. Don't let your success, progress, and process be contingent on anyone else's.

If you want to share, keep it simple; "I'm embarking on a food adventure, it's whole real foods, that's all." The more you try to explain it, the more they may find ways to talk you out of it, argue against it, guilt you out of it, shame you away from it, or pull out an arsenal of articles, books, posts, and memes to simply muck up your focus and intention.

Remember: People's responses are all about them. Not you. They react with their personal level of comfort, understanding, education, and emotional intelligence. Watching you explore, evolve and transition for the better will poke at all the places where they are not doing this for themselves. It's ok. Just let this journey be yours.

This process is about the capacity to feel amazing versus feeling at the mercy of your body. It's about working with our system in the way it's intended to function. It's about learning to have a constructive conversation with your body and continue the conversation, translation, and response in a healthy way throughout our life.

More often than not the Reset becomes about so much more than just cracking your personal food code. It becomes about breaking up with the dysfunctional emotional paradigms we have with food and social endeavors.

The Reset is powerful … yet soft in its approach. These realizations will be slow and sneaky, but powerful all the same.

You really don't have to do what everyone else is doing, you simply have to be bolstered in your resolve and know that it's ok for you to do, or eat, one thing and for someone else to do, or eat, another. Leave the judgment, yours and others, off the menu.

We are all uniquely different and each in our own place on the journey of life. Much as I wish for it, we just can't all be at the same place at the same time. It's your time to Reset. It may not be everyone else's.

Notes on Reset Foods

You can make and eat every meal that is listed below or you can pick and choose. For example choose one smoothie for your week of breakfasts. You do not have to do all three. You may also leave out the Coconut Yogurt if you cannot find the coconut kefir probiotics I recommend.

It's also ok to make only two soups or two proteins instead of all three. Take the time to read through the entire menu and mark off what you won't need from your grocery list if you are narrowing the menu or if you simply can't find the exact ingredients.

Notice above that I did not say to make substitutions, please do the Reset as written. There is no need to get creative, add, or modify anything. The Reset is written with great care to minimize digestive distress, allowing time for it to heal, be bolstered with the highest amount of nutrients possible in the shortest amount of time and give you the clearest possible answers to what does and does not work for your body in 41 days time.

The narrow menu and repetition are intentional. The Reset is not only an opportunity to crack your own food code and generate a health upswing, it's also an opportunity to break some major emotional and cultural bonds with food.

Think of the Reset as the capsule wardrobe of food. You have things that always work and always make you feel good that you don't have to put too much thought into for 41 days. It creates literal space to think of and about things other than food.

I love food. I love beautiful meals and I am all about experiencing life and the quality of it with creativity. However, the Reset is not the time for creative endeavors in food. It's time to heal, to learn, to explore and to evolve for the better. It's only 41 days. You have plenty of time to get creative with food post Reset.

The Reset is a huge opportunity to explore the pressures of social eating as well as disordered eating habits. Do we still get to celebrate and gather around a meal? Yes! Of course, but remember that gathering to celebrate a holiday or birthday is about the holiday or the person … not simply an excuse to gorge on food.

Embrace this food adventure as written. It works. Journal. Take notes. Talk to me and others that have completed or are currently completing the Reset in my private

Facebook group <u>The Reset</u>. Allow for the space of not knowing, feeling new and better, breaking false paradigms where food is concerned and generations of misunderstandings about nutrition dissipate.

The Reset is for everyone. You will always learn something from it. The Reset has particular healing power for those with known or suspected autoimmune issues but the majority of people need and require a health upswing that starts in the gut. The Reset is powerful. You'll finally crack your food code and be able to thrive minus the mystery. You'll get answers and results that last a lifetime rather than just 30, 60, or 90 days. And if you ever fall off your wellness wagon with food, you'll always know where to come back to to climb back on.

Most who do the Reset do it a minimum of three times. Practice makes proficient and repetition generates mastery. It takes time, but the Reset is well worth the journey.

Why Lamb

Over the years of all the questions I get about the Reset, one of the most frequently asked is "Why is lamb on the menu?" Poor little lambs, don't get enough appreciation. Lamb is the bloodiest of animal proteins. It's the best to support a female system because of our cycles and the typical, small bit of anemia we experience, especially during menstruation. Traditional Chinese Medicine speaks to this usage of it. It's a much healthier red meat with more iron and zinc than other animal proteins. It's packed with selenium and the biggie: B12. It's packed with all the good fats and you only need 3 ounces of lamb to reap the powerhouse benefits of its nutrient profile, and all the magical B12 supports energy levels while supporting your nervous system in an incredibly calming and balancing way. Lamb also packs a punch for bolstering your immune system.

Remember, the Reset is written to bolster, nourish, support, and heal your body. All the foods and cooking methods are chosen with great care to pack a punch with nutrient density and preservation or accessibility. The Reset menu is designed to be gentle on your digestive system while getting as many nutrients into your system in the shortest amount of time.

Although a full gut healing can take 12 to 24 months, the Reset is designed to give you an incredible boost to that healing while cracking your personal food code. The Reset menu lays the groundwork in a thoughtful and educated, yet accessible manner.

Fermented Foods

Most people nowadays have some understanding that fermented foods are good for them but may be unclear as to why they are good for you. The short answer is fermented foods like pickles, kimchi, sauerkraut, kombucha, and kefir, contain a plethora of good bacteria that help balance overall gut bacteria.

To have a truly healthy body you must get the gut bacteria balanced. The typical standard American diet (SAD) cultivates the bad bacteria, therefore your gut flora is out of balance. When the gut flora is out of balance it creates a home that disease and illness love to live in, like E.Coli and Salmonella. An imbalance of bad gut bacteria literally throws your mood way off.

Mood you say? It's not a complete farce that the way to happiness is through your stomach? Yup. Looks like our grandmothers were right to feed us in order to demonstrate love.

There are more serotonin receptors in your gut than there are in your brain. So this idea that we treat anxiety and depression via brain chemicals, is in of itself, imbalanced.

Fermented foods are a probiotic. Probiotics are *good* bacteria that balance your gut flora for it's healthiest baseline, best digestion and mood.

Kombucha and sauerkraut are chosen for the the Reset menu because they are the second and third most powerful fermented foods.

What's the first, you say, and why isn't it on the Reset? The first is kefir, but it's dairy-based and since dairy is on our "no" list initially it's not a universal *do-no-harm* food.

Kombucha is a fermented beverage packed with probiotics, B vitamins, vinegar, and enzymes that aid in digestion, weight loss and general detox. If you have trouble with kombucha make sure to check the label that it's only tea, sugar and perhaps a fruit or element such as ginger in it. Label reading is beyond important to your Reset experience and results. Not all kombuchas are created equally. Just like with any other food stay far away from natural flavors or natural flavoring or even citric acid.

Yes, it's okay for the sugar to be on the label, it's not actually in your kombucha. It's used in the brewing process to generate the good bacteria — the stuff swirling at the bottom of the jar — where all the good bacteria is. You're not actually drinking all the sugar that brewed the good bacteria, you're drinking what the chemical reaction between the sugar and black tea and scoby (mother bacteria that generates the process of growing the bacterial culture in kombucha).

You can brew your own kombucha at home. Homemade is always best but if you don't have the time or bandwidth to monitor its growth, store bought works just fine.

If you still have trouble with kombucha after checking the label, go smaller on your portions, start with 2 oz. at a time and work to 4 oz. or 6 oz. a day. You don't need more than that a day.

Sometimes the balance in your personal system is so far off the mark of balanced that it takes time to find the good balance with kombucha.

Sauerkraut is the third most beneficial fermented food. Sauerkraut is raw cabbage and sea salt in vinegar that has been allowed to ferment — fermentation is the chemical process of converting carbohydrates to alcohol — the ingredients are aged and allowed to brew. Fermentation happens in the process of making bread, cheese, olives, wine, beer, vinegar, and even yogurt. Though the process is a part of all of these foods, the quality or power of the fermentation is not the same throughout the list. Sauerkraut is packed with vitamins C and K, iron, and B vitamins. It's a powerhouse.

Fermented foods basically plant good bacteria bugs in your belly allowing for healing, a proper balance of gut bacteria and overall better digestion and nutrient absorption. They are a must for a fit and healthy system.

Tea

Hot tea is one of the sneakiest places that gluten hides. I know how strange this sounds but it's true. It's also a hotbed (pun intended) of other body-irritating junk. When it comes to tea on the Reset make sure you are investing in organic variations. Tea leaves are such a small surface area that are laden with chemicals to ward off pests. If tea is not organic, it's very often not even washed prior to the aging of the leaves.

You want organic tea leaves to ensure a clean source is going into your gorgeous body.

In addition to an organic label on your tea, you want to make sure there are no artificial flavorings or flavors in your cup. These are the secret hideaways of gluten, fake or chemical flavorings and or preservatives. The label of "flavor" or "flavoring" is essentially code for *anything-we-want-to-put-in-here.* It's added in such small amounts that the labeling laws allow it. I know your instant thought is: it's such a small amount that it shouldn't matter, I'm fine, I'm not sensitive, I'm not diagnosed with anything. This is where you are wrong, or potentially wrong. It's something you'll need to test post Reset for your body. For my body, it matters, I react to even the smallest amount. For my boys, it's often okay.

During the Reset, keep your sources of tea squeaky clean for best and uncompromised results. Post Reset do what works for your body.

Chicken and the Bone Broth

On the Reset it's best for your whole bird to be pasture raised, hormone- and antibiotic-free. Please don't buy a pre-roasted bird or go cheap on this one. The cleanliness of your bird matters, not only for your general meal but for the quality of your bone broth that you will make from the leftover bones.

Please do NOT buy premade bone broth. Though there are some wonderful variations of clean broth now available on the market, nutrient density is always better when it's homemade plus we are practising the honoring of the entire bird and using as much of it as we can.

On the Reset I recommend chicken bone broth as opposed to others sources because chicken bone broth has the highest content of collagen and therefore is the most healing to the gut lining.

Collagen from clean animal proteins is the only way to heal and seal damage to the gut lining — leaky gut. This is why there is not a vegan option to the Reset. In order to heal you must have the collagen. Bone broth is also packed with glucosamine, glutamine, calcium, and magnesium your body can easily digest. It's also a powerful support to your immune system.

Bone broth is one of the best examples of how whole real foods can supply all the nutritional elements and components we need in order to thrive if we get the right sources in place.

Coconut Water

Coconut water is a wonderful source of hydration and it is included in your smoothie recipes. It also has a decent amount of sugar, so, no you can't guzzle it all day. Stick to water and tea for your Reset. Keep the coconut water to your smoothies and the carrot soup.

Fruit

Questions about fruit are another of the most frequently asked questions about the Reset. Can I eat more fruit? Can I eat the fruit listed on the menu as much as I want, at any time of day?

No. Nope. No.

One of the main benefits of the Reset is that you can truly break up with sugar addictions and cravings by completing your Reset.

Fruit is a wonderful source of nutrients, fiber, and alkalinity for our bodies. However, fruit isn't intended to be the bulk of our nutritional sources. It's meant to complement our overall nutrient profiles … but we are not meant to live by fruit alone.

The truth of the matter is that fruit is sugar. Fruit is gorgeous and full of good stuff, but when it gets inside our bodies, it's also sugar. Bodies cannot distinguish where glucose or fructose come from, only that they are there. It's unbelievably important to minimize the amount of sugars inside the body for the baseline of your healing, fitness, and wellness process.

Our bodies get addicted to sweet, to the sugar. Regardless of where it is sourced from. The only way to cut a sugar addiction or sugar craving is to drastically cut our consumption or completely starve it out.

Sugars feed on sugar. You've heard it over and over again that people cannot eat any sugar lest they open the floodgates to the entire sugar demon. Once they start, they cannot stop.

In the initial healing stages, we all need to starve out our sugars. In order to truly cultivate gut flora balance between good and bad bacteria, we need to keep the sugars low, low, low.

Fruit is minimally included in your smoothies because they offer cooling and alkalizing properties to the body from a Traditional Chinese Medicine perspective, they offer wonderful antioxidants for vibrant health, fiber plus a bit of hydration. Your body does require glucose and fructose to optimally run, it just doesn't want an overload.

This is a major mishap most people make when they are attempting to *eat healthy* — I have a grand dislike for that phrase. Eating healthy is not odd, it's the way we are designed to eat. It's just eating in accordance to our physical design. People will reach for fruit and call it healthy — and it *is* better — but it's not the answer. Those who reach for fruit and never touch a vegetable are totally missing the wellness boat. Balance is always the answer and cracking your personal food code is the ultimate wellness.

If you find yourself craving fruit and immediately wanting to add more to your Reset — stop — refer back to section where I said not to modify, add or adjust the Reset menu unless you already know certain foods trigger bad things in your body. The Reset is not a creative endeavor. If you're craving fruit, you know you've got a sugar monster to manage, and you've got a relationship with sweets you'll be reviewing, adjusting, and evolving past in these 41 days.

Sweet tastes are wired as reward in our body. They are typically emotional. Sweet and sugar, regardless of the source, is not where we want the bulk of our fuel to come from.

In order to truly break up with a sugar addiction you'll need to address the fruit side of things as well. Sugar disrupts your insulin levels, insulin levels directly affect your energy levels and your capacity to lose weight. Honor the fruit minimization on this food adventure and I promise it'll have you thriving like never before.

Insulin is a hormone. Your ultimate wellness in your physical body relies on hormone balance. Insulin could be pointed to as the biggest player in this equation. Honor this. If you stabilize and balance your insulin by being conscious and aware of your sugars, even from fruit, you'll reap the rewards in no time!

Enjoy the fruit included on the Reset. Keep it to the morning and keep it in your smoothies. Allow your cravings to be snuffed out in these 41 days. Post Reset explore more wonderful fruits and see how your system responds.

Lemon Water

Warm lemon water in the morning is a simple and powerful cleanser for your internal system. It flushes the liver daily for an overall smooth running cleanse plus it boosts your metabolism because it cleanses your liver.

Every morning of your Reset, begin with a cup of four to eight ounces of warm water with half a lemon squeezed in it. Keep it real — no you can't use lemon essential oil, though it is similar, it's not the same as a real lemon. The Reset is all about getting back to and keeping things real. There is a grounding element to the Reset as well because we focus on touching, connecting and consuming real food, as it is, from the earth. The Reset is sooooo not about shortcuts.

Drinking warm lemon water can be a finicky thing like drinking kombucha. If you've never done it before your system may respond with a bit of heartburn or acid reflux. This is one of the particular instances, like kombucha, where the reaction is not a signal to stop doing it, it's a signal of how badly your body needs it.

Alkaline foods flush your system for the better and the healthier. An alkaline environment discourages bacteria and disease from brewing. It's not an absolute prevention to health issues, but it's as close as we can get to it.

Lemons are highly alkaline for your internal system. They are acidic on the pH scale outside of our bodies … but when they are inside our digestive tract, they are alkaline. Behold the wonders of science!

If you have reactions like heartburn or acid reflux with the warm lemon water in the morning, like kombucha, back off of the amount of lemon to a quarter of a fresh lemon for one to two weeks, then work your way back up.

Yes, you can add lemon to your water all day long for general hydration if you would like to, while on the Reset.

The Reset does speak to an overall alkaline diet. Plant based is the way to go, but as we covered prior, plant-based means 85-95% plant-based. Your diet does not have to be 100% alkaline in order to be on the alkaline scale for optimal wellness. Balance is key in all things. Cracking your own food code is imperative to know how much acid your particular body can handle.

Supplements and Medications

I've never been an advocate for supplements or vitamins. Our bodies are designed to pull and process and receive nutrients from whole real foods, not from processed pills or powders. Supplements tax your liver and just end up being expensive urine. Whole real foods supply everything we need. We simply have to supply those elements for our body and have a body well enough to function, pull, and process those nutrients.

Take yourself off as many supplements, over-the-counter medications and potentially medications — **only IF it is okayed with your doctor(s)** — prior to embarking on the Reset.
Medications are a huge source of gut damage and overall health issues that we don't realize.
Medications are something we ingest … we are eating them … medications are packed with fillers and binders that are often our very source of pain, inflammation, symptoms, and reactions. These fillers and binders can include gluten, corn, dairy, nightshades (mostly potato starch), and soy.

I speak from personal experience on this one.

Clean out what you can during your Reset. Manage small headaches or body aches and pains with rest, water, epsom salt baths, and essential oils. The big stuff you cannot come off of just yet … honor it … embark on the Reset and allow it to be the #betterisbetter concept. Doing the Reset even while on your medications that potentially have fillers that cause problems will still generate an upswing and will lead you down the path to more empowered knowledge and will allow you to keep walking the path to wellness post Reset. You will still be able to pinpoint what gives you major trouble … you just might not feel as amazing as you will once you can switch to a medication that doesn't have your trigger in it. The long term goal would be to eventually heal to the place where you no longer require meds or can be off of most of them.

I no longer have a thyroid. I am on daily medication for the rest of my life. Three years post surgery I found an option for a medication that doesn't have any of my triggers in it.

Healing happens.
Don't give up hope.

Don't give up seeking.
Be diligent and warrior for yourself and your best health.
Allow for better … because better feels unbelievably amazing.

Do what you can without getting caught up in perfection for your Reset. Be aware, allow space for better, than dig into the minutia of details post-Reset if you aren't feeling utterly amazing already.

The Power of Food

The power and healing capacity of food is sorely underestimated and highly undervalued. If you only ever read the Reset, you'll learn something about yourself, the power of food and your emotional bonds with it.

Every time you do the Reset, no matter how much of it you complete, you'll learn something valuable about your body and its relationship with food. Any time with the

Reset is time well spent for your wellness and relationship with your physical body.

Post Reset

Don't give up on the Reset or eating clean simply because it's day 41.

Stick with whole real foods. Don't waste all the effort you just gave for 41 days by capsizing on sweet/fruit, or junk, convenient, or comfort food. Remember the Reset is not a diet. It's a discovery of what foods work for you and not against you for your best health.

The Reset is meant to crack your personal food code for your thrival and best life experience. It's not something to quickly discard and toss aside.
Salads and clean proteins are always a good idea, as is staying away from processed foods and treats etc. Full hydration and minimal caffeine or alcohol are always winners.

Don't add too many new things in one day after your Reset.
Your system will not be happy with you.

Honor the effort you've put in and the information you've gained thus far and anchor into what you've learned. Your intuition and how your body responds to things is pure wellness gold. Take a bit of time post Reset to sit and sort through your journal and how you feel is best to transition in the days following day 41.

You have more answers and solutions than you realize. Ask yourself what you think is best within the rails of your original goal of embarking on the Reset: health, healing, wellness, fitness, travel, fun, joy, and life in general.

Don't be so quick to run off the rails. Don't rush back to emotional distancing or rewarding with your fuel. What have you learned? What do you think about in terms of food and fuel now that you didn't before? How do you feel now versus how you felt when you began? How do you want to continue to feel more days than not in your life? Are you committed to your wellness and to your best self? Are you still tied to what seems easier or what everyone else is doing? Are you committed to health care prevention and healing? Or are you ok with symptom management and looming long-term health issues down the road? How do you want to show up in the world and will you allow your fuel to support and generate the best version of that?

Clearly there's a world of gorgeous and wonderful foods we didn't test in the Reset. Take your time to see if they work for you or not. Be aware. Stay connected and in conversation with your body. Try the things you missed most or that make your life more efficient first ... and again, don't pile three or four new elements in in one day. That's just mean to your system after all the nurturing, caring, and bolstering you've done for it.

You provide so much self-love for your body, mind, and spirit during the Reset! I'm proud of you for being adventurous, open and brave! Thank you for being willing to transform and heal.

RESET MENU	DAY 1	DAY 2	DAY 3	DAY 4	DAY 5
MORNING	PUMPKIN JUICE	GREEN RESET SMOOTHIE	BERRY RESET SMOOTHIE	GREEN RESET SMOOTHIE	BERRY RESET SMOOTHIE
AM SNACK	PROBIOTIC SNACK	PROBIOTIC SNACK	PROBIOTIC SNACK	PROBIOTIC SNACK	PROBIOTIC SNACK
LUNCH	ROAST CHICKEN W/ VEGGIES OR GREENS	RESET SALAD #1	BASIL GINGER SALMON W/ VEGGIES	RESET SALAD #2	RESET SALAD #3
PM SNACK	1 CUP OF TEA + 2 TBSP COCONUT BUTTER	1 CUP OF TEA + VEGGIES W/ PESTO	1 CUP OF TEA + 2 TBSP COCONUT BUTTER	1 CUP OF TEA + VEGGIES W/ PESTO	1 CUP OF TEA + 2 TBSP COCONUT BUTTER
DINNER	RESET CARROT SOUP + FLOUNDER	RESET GREEN SOUP + CHICKEN	RESET CARROT SOUP + VEGGIES	RESET GREEN SOUP + FISH	RESET BEET SOUP + LAMB PATTIES
TEA	1 CUP OF TEA ½ HOUR BEFORE BED	1 CUP OF TEA ½ HOUR BEFORE BED	1 CUP OF TEA ½ HOUR BEFORE BED	1 CUP OF TEA ½ HOUR BEFORE BED	1 CUP OF TEA ½ HOUR BEFORE BED

Breakfast Smoothies

Pumpkin Juice

In a blender combine:
- 1 cup organic pumpkin puree (out of a can works and is what I do)
- 2 cups coconut water
- 1 small banana
- 1 teaspoon cinnamon
- add water to adjust the consistency if you need to

Reset Green Smoothie

In a blender combine:
- 1 cup kale

- 1 cup spinach
- ½ of an avocado
- 2 cups coconut water
- add water to adjust the consistency if you need to

Berry Reset Smoothie

In a blender combine:
- 1 banana
- 2 cups coconut water
- ½ cup organic cherries (frozen or fresh)
- 1 cup mixed organic berries (fresh or frozen, blueberry, raspberry and strawberry blend)
- add water to adjust the consistency if you need to

****BONUS RECIPE #1 - HOT CACAO****
ONLY after Day 26 if all the ingredients work for your system.
Ingredients:
- 2 tablespoons organic, raw cacao nibs
- 1 teaspoon raw honey

- 1/2 teaspoon of Ceylon Cinnamon
  Yes, Ceylon. It matters … not just
  any cinnamon will do for the healing
  and nutritional properties.
- 8 oz. of hot water or clean coconut
  milk — Clean means no additives
  and most particularly no guar gum.
  Using dairy milk negates most of the
  benefits of the cacao as it hinders
  absorption. I use ½ cup of hot water
  from a tea kettle and ½ cup coconut
  milk.

Directions:
Blend all ingredients in a blender until all
the cacao nibs are no longer nibs. Pour in
a mug and enjoy!

BONUS RECIPE #2 - HEMP MILK
ONLY on or after Day 15
Ingredients:
- 1 cup shelled organic hemp seeds
- 4 cups water
- a pinch of pink salt

Directions:

Combine the ingredients in a blender until smooth. Once the mixture is smooth, pour it through a cheesecloth, nut bag, or a clean pair of nylons or a strainer to filter out the "chunks." I do this twice and usually in a strainer when I do hemp milk.

Pour into a container and store in fridge for up to seven days.

Post Reset, if you like, you add a vanilla bean to it and let it soak in the milk.

After you've tested sugars, Day 26-28: If your system tolerates raw honey or pure maple syrup you can add a teaspoon of either to this recipe for added sweetness.

Mid-Morning Snack

Each day for a mid-morning snack, choose one of the following:

- **2 - 6 oz. of Kombucha** (store bought or homemade) Make sure to read the labels. Avoid all artificial and natural flavorings. The sugar listed in Kombucha is fine, it's used in the fermentation, to grow the food bacteria. It's not actually present in what you are consuming. No Kombucha with chia or spirulina in it. I recommend GT's Kombucha and am in no way sponsored by them, It's the most common to come by and the cleanest.
- **1 - 3 tablespoons Sauerkraut** that is fermented in brine water (water and salt) only or brine water and vinegar — no nightshades, no herbs or seasoning.
- **1/2 - 1 cup Homemade Coconut Yogurt** This one is so simple it's almost embarrassing. Mix an entire can of clean organic coconut milk — check the label for only coconut milk, coconut creme, and water. Absolutely no guar gum, additives, or thickeners — with 1 tablespoon of Inner-Eco Fresh Coconut Water Probiotic in a

clean jar and place in your oven with only the light on for 24 hours. It will not *set up* like yogurt that we are used to. It's runny and tangy. It's *yogurt* because it's fermented with probiotics.

This is something you can cut from your Reset menu if you're not interested or cannot find the listed ingredients. However, if dairy ends up not working for you it's a lovely, creamy substitute.

Lunch

Lunches include salads and lean proteins — roast chicken, salmon, or lamb burger patties — with any of your batch cooked or raw veggies on your grocery list.

Dress your salads simply with any combo of the following: fresh lemon, orange, blood orange, or lime juice, and olive oil.

Remember, this is a Reset for your palate and stomach, go simple.

Reset Salad #1

- arugula, romaine or iceberg lettuce or any combo of the three
- baked sweet potato
- roasted or raw beets
- sautéed or raw baby bella mushrooms
- Any of your batch cooked proteins: roast chicken, salmon, flounder, or lamb patty

Reset Salad #2

- arugula, romaine or iceberg lettuce or any combo of the three
- roasted parsnips, carrots
- raw sliced radishes
- raw chopped celery
- Any of your batch cooked proteins: roast chicken, flounder, salmon, or lamb patty

Reset Salad #3

- arugula, romaine or iceberg lettuce or any combo of the three

- roasted or raw carrots and roasted sweet potatoes
- Any of your batch cooked proteins: roast chicken, salmon, flounder, or lamb patty

See Batch Cooking Instructions for:
- **Roast Chicken**
- **Basil Ginger Salmon**
- **Lamb Burger Patties**
- **Flounder**

Midday Snack

Tea is a fab easy way to help flush toxins from your system.
During your Reset I recommend up to three servings of organic herbal tea per day. One cup in the first half of the day, a cup in the afternoon, and perhaps one cup before bed.

Choose one or all flavors during your Reset:
- Peppermint
- Ginger
- Turmeric

- Tulsi

Be diligent about reading the labels, no additives to your tea, just simple, clear ingredients.

Each afternoon, if you're hungry, enjoy a cup of tea and one of the following:

- 1-3 tablespoons coconut butter — straight outta the jar is how I do it.
- Any of your batch cooked or raw veggies, mushrooms or greens: arugula, romaine, iceberg lettuce, beet greens, dandelion greens in whatever amount satiates your afternoon hunger. Listen to your body and respond to what it's telling you each afternoon. Keep your small amounts of kale or spinach to your smoothie only.

Veggie choices in the afternoon include: cauliflower, broccoli, asparagus, carrots, parsnips, beets, sweet potatoes, Brussels sprouts, and yellow or green zucchini and cucumber — yes, cucumber is technically a fruit it is allowed on the Reset.

- Raw carrots, radish, celery, green or yellow zucchini, or cucumbers with Reset Pesto — recipe below.

Reset Pesto

Ingredients:
- 4 cups fresh basil
- 1 cup fresh tarragon
- 1/4 cup unfiltered olive oil — You can use any olive oil but unfiltered has the most benefit. If you need to add a little more or even less oil for your blender or preference, you can.

Directions:
In a food processor or blender, combine until smooth.

Dinner

Dinners each day include Reset Soups, lean proteins, and lots of veggies. Recipes for the following dinner items can be found in the batch cooking instruction area.

Reset Soups
- Reset Carrot Soup
- Reset Green Soup
- Reset Beet Soup

Reset Proteins
- Roast Chicken
- Basil Ginger Salmon
- Lamb Burger Patties
- Flounder

Reset Veggies
- Greens: arugula, romaine, iceberg lettuce, beet greens or dandelion greens
- Cauliflower
- Cucumber
- Broccoli
- Asparagus
- Carrots
- Parsnips
- Beets
- Sweet potatoes
- Brussels sprouts

- Green zucchini
- Mushrooms
- Raw carrots
- Raw radishes
- Celery

General Guidelines

I encourage you to add as many veggies to all snacks and meals as you need to. If you are hungry, eat. If you aren't particularly hungry try to at least eat what is listed for you. Listen to your body. Cultivate connection and awareness to what it needs, at each point in the day and honor that.

During the Reset I have you cooking a lot of food so it's there if you need it. **Do not go hungry.** You may find at the end of the Reset you have leftovers — share or freeze them. If you need to pack things to go for work, make sure you have containers ready and pre-packed for the week.

HYDRATION GOAL for the Reset — In general you should consume half your bodyweight in ounces of water daily. Hydration is huge for body results, capacity to absorb and process the amount of fiber on your menu, energy levels, and true wellness. You need it to flush out toxins and waste.

Please make your hydration a priority on the Reset.

Begin every morning, prior to any eating or drinking, have 4-8 oz of warm water with the juice of half of a fresh lemon.

Batch Cooking: Veggies

Gather all of the produce on the list below that you need for your chosen recipes:

- 8 sweet potatoes — my favorite are the Japanese variety.

- 2-3 boxes of baby bella or button mushrooms or 4-6 cups - no other varieties
- 5-6 large parsnips
- 5 lb. bag of carrots
- 1 head of cauliflower
- 1 lb. Brussels sprouts
- 8 medium beets
- 1 Bosc pear
- 4 green or yellow zucchini
- 5 lemons
- 1 large baking dish
- Parchment paper
- 3- 4 cookie sheets or baking dishes for your veggies
- 2 tablespoon olive oil
- large saute pan
- 3 tablespoons of coconut oil
- Himalayan pink salt
- Fresh cracked pepper

Directions:

- Wash all veggies and fruit. Cut up raw veggies as you like and place them in containers in the refrigerator for use during the week. Reserve as many of the carrots for eating raw as you like, saving about half the bag for the soup and the remainder roasted.

- Preheat your oven to 350 degrees.
- Place skin-on sweet potatoes, beets, asparagus, pear, and cut up cauliflower in separate baking dishes or cookie sheets.
- Peel your carrots and parsnips and place them in an oven-safe baking dish together. Slather them in coconut oil and sprinkle with pink salt (up to a teaspoon). Mix thoroughly to spread oil and salt evenly over all veggies. Cover with parchment paper. Parchment paper versus aluminum foil minimizes toxic load on the body.
- Roast all of the above in the oven for 1 ½ hours.
- Chop mushrooms into small pieces.
- Heat 1 tablespoon of olive oil in a large pan over medium heat on the stove. Add mushrooms, pink salt, and fresh ground pepper to taste. Sauté, stirring periodically, for approximately 5-8 minutes or until you see the

mushrooms start to shrink down. Remove from pan.

- Cut your Brussels sprouts in half. Add 1 tablespoon olive oil to the same pan you used for the mushrooms, add your Brussels sprouts, salt, pepper, and the juice of one lemon and sauté for approximately 10 minutes. Remove from pan.
- Slice zucchini any length or width you desire. Add 1 tablespoon olive oil to the same pan, add your cut zucchini, salt, pepper, and the juice of one lemon and sauté for approximately 5-8 minutes.

Batch Cooking: Proteins

ROAST CHICKEN

Ingredients:
- 1 whole organic chicken
- 1 lemon
- 1/2 an orange

- 1/2 cup of any of the following fresh herbs: basil, rosemary, sage, thyme, or tarragon
- 1 tablespoon coconut or olive oil
- pink salt and fresh pepper to taste

Directions:
- Preheat oven to 350-400 degrees.
- Take the whole bird and place it in a baking dish.
- Slather it in approximately 1 tablespoon of olive oil or coconut oil and any mixture of seasoning you wish (rosemary is my fave but fresh basil and oregano work as well).
- Squeeze the juice of 1/2 an orange and 1 lemon over the entire thing
- Stuff the citrus rinds inside the bird.
- Leave uncovered, place in oven for approximately 2 hours.
- Save the bones from your roast chicken to make Bone Broth for soup recipes.

BASIL GINGER SALMON

Ingredients:

- 1 pound wild caught salmon
- 1/2 cup fresh basil, chopped
- 1 teaspoon dried ginger
- 1 lemon
- 1 tablespoon coconut oil
- pink salt and fresh pepper to taste

Directions:

- In a pan over medium heat on the stove, add the coconut oil and half of your basil leaves and half of your ginger to the bottom of the pan.
- Add the salmon, skin down.
- Sprinkle the remaining basil and ginger over the top of the salmon.
- Cook undisturbed until you see half of your salmon turn a lighter shade of pink, approximately 5 minutes, then flip it over.
- Continue to cook until done, approximately another 5-8 minutes.
- Remove and serve or store.

LAMB BURGER PATTIES

Ingredients:

- 1 lb. organic ground lamb

- 1 cup fresh sage, thyme, and rosemary, chopped and mixed to equal a cup
- pink salt and fresh pepper to taste

Directions:

- In a large bowl mix your lamb and your herbs.
- Divide and shape four patties.
- Place in an oven-safe dish, uncovered in the oven.
- Bake at 325 degrees for 20-25 minutes.

RESET FLOUNDER – If you can't find flounder, cod makes a nice substitute

Ingredients:

- 2 flounder fillets
- 1 tablespoon coconut oil
- 1 lemon
- pink salt and fresh pepper to taste

Directions:

- Melt coconut oil in a pan over medium heat on the stove.

- Add your fillets, with salt and pepper to taste.
- Cook approximately 3 minutes then flip and add fresh lemon juice. Cook another 3 minutes, then serve.

Batch Cooking: Soups

CHICKEN BONE BROTH

Ingredients:
- the leftover bones of 1 roasted chicken
- pink salt to taste
- 2 bay leaves
- 2 tablespoons of apple cider vinegar

Directions:
- Place a large soup pot on the stove.
- Add everything to the pot, then fill it 3/4 of the way with water.
- Cover and bring to a boil.
- Then bring it down to a rolling simmer and let it simmer for as long as you can (four to 12 hours).

- When you are ready to pull it off the heat, pour it through a strainer, discard the solids, and use the flavorful broth for your soup.

You can freeze any extra and save the golden element for later use.

RESET GREEN SOUP

Ingredients:
- 2 bags frozen organic broccoli
- 1 shallot
- 1 tablespoon olive oil
- 4-6 cups **Bone Broth** (substitute whatever broth works for you, but bone broth has the most healing potential for a gut).

Directions:
- In large saucepan or soup pot on the stove over medium heat, saute the shallot in olive oil until translucent.
- Add the broccoli and bone broth. Bring to a boil.

- Boil until veggies are soft, approximately 10 minutes.
- Transfer everything on the stove to a blender.
- Blend until smooth.

RESET CARROT SOUP

Ingredients:
- 1 tablespoon coconut oil
- 1 shallot, chopped
- About 12 medium-sized carrots, peeled and chopped
- 2 cups coconut water
- 1/4 teaspoon pink salt
- 1/4 teaspoon sage powder
- 1/4 teaspoon dried ginger

Directions:
- In a large saucepan or soup pot on the stove over medium heat, melt the coconut oil and sauté the shallot until translucent. Add in the sage and dried ginger and allow to saturate and warm up in the coconut oil for a minute.

- Add the carrots and coconut water. Bring to a boil.
- Boil until carrots are soft, approximately 15 minutes.
- Transfer everything on the stove to a blender.
- Blend until smooth.

RESET BEET SOUP

Ingredients:
- 5 medium beets – pre roasted from your batch cooking
- 5 sprigs fresh tarragon
- 4 cups **Bone Broth** (substitute whatever broth works for you, but bone broth has the most healing potential for a gut).
- 1 Bosc pear — pre-roasted from your batch cooking
- pink salt

Directions:
- Peel the beets and pear when done baking (either straight from the oven or later during the week from the fridge).

- Combine all ingredients in blender. If you prepare this later in the week after you've roasted your beets and pear you'll need to heat it on the stove after you blend it.
- Blend until smooth.

Reset Grocery List

___ 8 Sweet Potatoes

___ 2-3 boxes Mushrooms — baby bella or button mushrooms only

___ 5-6 large Parsnips

___ 5 lb. bag of Carrots

___ 1 head of Cauliflower

___ 1 lb. Brussels Sprouts

___ 8 Red Beets

___ 4 Green and/or Yellow zucchini

___ 1 Avocado

___ 2 Shallots — no large onions, shallots only

___ 12 cups/servings Fresh Greens — may include: arugula, beet greens, dandelion greens, romaine or iceberg lettuce

___ any Fresh Radishes

___ 1 bunch Celery

___ 1 Cucumber

___ 6-10 Lemons

___ 1 Orange or Blood Orange

___ 1 Bosc Pear

___ 3 Bananas

___ 2 cups organic Mixed Berries (fresh or frozen blueberry, raspberry and strawberry blend)

___ 1 cup organic Cherries (frozen or fresh)

___ 6 cups Fresh Basil

___ 1 bunch Fresh Tarragon

___ 1 bunch Fresh Rosemary

___ 1 bunch Fresh Thyme

___ 1 bunch Fresh Sage

___ 1 Whole Organic Pasture-raised Chicken

___ 1 lb. Wild-Caught Salmon

___ 2 Wild-caught Flounder fillets or Cod if you cannot find flounder

___ 1 lb. Ground Lamb

___ Organic Tea — ginger, peppermint, tulsi, or turmeric

___ 2-3 16-oz. bottles of Kombucha

___ 2 large cartons of Organic, Unsweetened Coconut Water

__ 1 can of clean Organic Coconut Milk — coconut milk, coconut creme, and water only

__ 1 container Inner-Eco Fresh Coconut Water Probiotic

__ 1 jar Organic Coconut Butter

__ 1 jar Unrefined Organic Coconut Oil

__ Unfiltered Organic Olive Oil — If you can't find this any olive oil will work.

__ 1 small bottle of Apple Cider Vinegar

__ 1 jar Sauerkraut

__ 1 can or box Organic Pumpkin Puree

__ 2 cups frozen Organic Spinach — only for the smoothies

__ 2 cups frozen Organic Kale — only for smoothies

__ 2 bags Frozen Broccoli

__ Himalayan Pink Salt

__ Fresh Cracked Pepper

__ Ground Ceylon Cinnamon — don't buy just any cinnamon

__ Ground Sage

__ Dried Ginger

__ Bay Leaves

__ Parchment Paper

Here's to your gut health, finding out what foods work for your body and your health and fitness results! You're brave for embarking on it and I'm already proud of you for being courageous enough to warrior for your own health, fitness, and wellness!

About the Author

Tandy Gutierrez is an internationally recognized educator in the fitness & wellness industry. She is the Creator and Head Unicorn of www.unicornwellnessstudio.com, an online studio that is a wellness home for members in over 50 countries since 2013. She is the creator and author of the 30 Days to Better online courses. She has honed a unique style of body, mind and spirit wellness that is intelligent, loving, intuitive, pure magic and healing.

Her work has been featured in Elle, Seventeen and Allure magazines and is consistently ranked one of the top Pilates instructors in the U.S. Tandy's clients include a roster of celebrities, professional dancers, Olympians, NFL, MLB, and Iron Man athletes and everyone in between and was the first Regional Director of Pilates for Equinox Fitness in Southern California.

Tandy has appeared in workouts for ExerciseTV, on-demand via cable providers nationwide and online. She has a diverse movement background from a full Pilates mat and apparatus certification, an NSCA CPT, martial arts, yoga and BFAs in Acting and Dance that she draws from in order to create intelligent and balanced workouts that prevent and heal injuries.

With nearly two decades in the fitness & wellness industry and 20+ years with the Pilates method she's known for igniting healing in the body issues no one else can make progress with.

Her personal journey with multiple chronic issues, injuries, pregnancies, IBS, Celiac, and a thyroidectomy has gifted her with an education on the power of self-care, simplicity and magic.